W9-AIJ-975

# ATLAS OF
# Breast
# Pathology

Folke Linell and Otto Ljungberg

# ATLAS OF
# Breast
# Pathology

Munksgaard
*Copenhagen*

*North and South America:*
J. B. Lippincott
*Philadelphia*

Atlas of Breast Pathology

Cover by Lars Thorsen
Typesetting: Satsform, Åbyhøj
Reproduction: Odense Reproduktion, Odense
Printed in Denmark 1984 by Th. Laursen, Tønder

ISBN 87-16-09636-3

**Distributed in North and South America by**
**J. B. Lippincott, Philadelphia**

ISBN 0-397-58297-3

**Library of Congress catalog card No. 85-50376**

# Acknowledgments

A work as this is impossible to carry out without close cooperation with clinical colleagues. The authors would like especially to thank Drs. Ingvar Andersson and Baldur Sigfusson, Department of Radiology, Drs. Ulf Ljungkvist, Knut Aspegren and Björn Sjöström, Department of Surgery, Drs. Björn Palmer and Anita Ringberg, Department of Plastic Surgery, Drs. Stig Borgström, Per Langeland and Torsten Landberg, Department of Oncology and Drs. Karin Lindholm and Lennart Bondeson, Department of Clinical Cytology. We also thank our colleagues at the Department of Pathology. Special thanks goes to the pathologists from other hospitals, who have contributed interesting cases. These are Drs. Kersti Hedberg, Kristianstad, Görel Östberg, Halmstad, Sweden, William and Henrik Kiaer, Svendborg, Denmark and Drs. Willebrand and V. Swaen, Maastricht, the Netherlands.

When this book was written and the pictures collected Dr. Fritz Rank, Copenhagen, read all the text and carefully scrutinized the photographs. For his critical remarks and positive suggestions for improvements we thank him warmly.

We also thank Mrs. Eva Minton, Monica Wetter, Lena Lundh and Leni Grubb, who have, with great skill, performed most of the histotechnical work, as well as Bengt Wängelin for invaluable photographic assistance. We are particularly indebted to Mrs. Inger Ahlström for the excellent typing and retyping of our manuscripts.

*Folke Linell / Otto Ljungberg*

# Preface

The purpose of this color atlas is primarily to serve as a help in the interpretation of breast lesions. It is principally aimed at the experienced pathologist, specialized in the field of breast pathology as well as the all-round pathologist, who receives a rather large proportion of breast specimens in his daily diagnostic practice. The book may also be of value as supplementary reading for medical students. We hope that it may be of interest to clinical colleagues working within other disciplines of medicine, such as diagnostic radiology, surgery and oncology, who, in their daily medical practice, are responsible for the management of patients with breast lesions. Hopefully, the book, in this way, may deepen the understanding between pathologists and their clinical colleagues.

Breast lesions represent a very important section of surgical pathology. Approximately ¼ of all female carcinomas are localized in the breasts. In addition, the breasts may develop a number of lesions which are important mainly in the differential diagnosis from carcinoma.

Mammography and other new developments of clinical diagnostic means have increased our knowledge of breast pathology immensely during the last 20 years. Great interest has been focused on the small carcinomas and their early, precancerous stages. These lesions have previously been ignored or considered of little clinical importance. Formerly when only large carcinomas were diagnosed by the one available method, palpation, the histologic diagnostics were very easy, but nowadays the early stages of carcinoma pose large problems to the pathologists.

Today, excision of a breast tumor not only aims at a histopathologic diagnosis of the lesion. The excised tumor is also used for assay of hormone receptor content and analysis of DNA-profiles, factors which may be of prognostic significance. The techniques employed for these studies are not dealt with in this book.

It should be stressed that fine needle aspiration biopsy has considerably contributed to the recent progress in the preoperative clinical diagnosis of breast tumors. The cytologic diagnosis of aspirated material from breast lesions, however, does not fall within the scope of this book. Excellent recent books in this field are available (see additional reading).

In recent years, a large number of joint trials for breast cancer therapy have been started. Such trials are of little value unless the principles for histopathologic diagnosis and classification used are uniform. We hope that this book will contribute towards attaining this uniformity.

We have been engaged in surgical pathology for 40 years and 20 years, respectively, and during the last 7-8 years we have personally handled all breast specimens at a large hospital. This material comprises more than 1000 carcinomas and a great number of breast specimens with other lesions. In addition, we have acquired valuable experience from specimens sent in for evaluation from the laboratories of other hospitals. The results found in a 3-year material of breast carcinomas have been published previously (Linell, Ljungberg & Andersson 1980). Some new concepts were presented in that publication. In the present atlas these concepts are related to other, current classifications and opinions. For an easier comparison we have in the atlas given in brackets the WHO nomenclature in the few cases, where it differs from our designations. Thus, the atlas may also be useful to readers who do not fully agree with our views. In the atlas we also present some new, original observations, not previously published.

The present book has two main sections. One part contains a brief text survey, and the other is a series of photographic illustrations in color.

The text section contains 10 chapters.

The text chapters are by necessity very short and do not enter into deep discussions. They aim to give a short survey of the lesions presented in the second part of the book, the color atlas. In the color atlas we have endeavored to collect most of the information in the text opposite the pictures. It is our hope that the atlas can be used as a benchbook in which the diagnosing pathologist can easily find examples (often many) of different lesions.

The lesions are presented in the same order as in the preceding text section. In order to facilitate the practical use of the book the chapters in this part have been divided into several subtitles. The legends to the pictures have been placed on the page opposite the picture. The text and the photographs have been selected not only to demonstrate characteristic "textbook" cases, but also – within the space limits given – to illustrate variations in histologic and cytologic features. These variations are frequently encountered in pathologic diagnostic work and often represent diagnostic pitfalls. We show many lesions at low magnification because it is frequently of major importance for a correct diagnosis to get a picture of the entire lesion. In such cases details of special interest are illustrated at higher magnification in neighboring pictures.

Among the variants described are some curious cases about which our knowledge is limited. The intention of such descriptions is to direct the spotlight on rare but distinct cases in the hope that other pathologists may discover additional examples, thus providing us with more information about the nature of these lesions.

The bibliography does not claim to be complete but should serve as an introduction to the literature.

# Contents

# PART TWO: COLOR ATLAS OF BREAST PATHOLOGY

*Part One*

# Text Survey

# Chapter 1

# The Technique of Macro- and Microscopic Study of Breast Specimens

The macroscopic examination of surgical breast specimens is a very important procedure in the diagnosis of breast lesions and has become even more vital nowadays when diagnosis is frequently dependent on very small lesions. It should be self-evident that this requires a diligent examination of the specimen by an experienced pathologist. With frozen sections this, of course, is even more important.

An adequate fixation of the specimen is of great importance for a correct histologic interpretation of breast lesions. Bad fixation causes loosening of cells from their surroundings, lumina of ducts and acini become filled with detached epithelial cells and cytologic detail is lost. This interferes with the correct interpretation of early histologic lesions, especially premalignant changes and carcinoma in situ lesions. The correct diagnosis of such lesions has become much more important today when many cases of breast cancer are detected at a very early stage, due to effective clinical screening procedures. Nevertheless, even if fixation has been properly performed, disturbing artifacts such as detachment of the stroma from the epithelial structures may sometimes develop. In this book, where all illustrations are derived from routine sections such artifacts cannot be completely avoided. This applies also to artifacts which may occur during sectioning or other procedures. Some of these seem to be

constant phenomena with the methods used and occasionally some, such as wrinkling and folding of the central parts of radial scars, may even serve as valuable diagnostic features. Paraffin sections are uneven in thickness and stretching. Therefore not all parts of a histological photograph are in ideal focus. Examples of this may be found in the figures.

Excisional specimens, more than 1 cm across, should be incised to ensure good penetration of the fixative (preferably 10% neutral formalin) and pieces of paper towel preferably placed in the incisions. Surgical specimens with small lesions detected at mammography should be pinned up on a plate and the lesions properly marked by the surgeon (or by the radiologist in cases where specimen radiography has been performed).

Mastectomy specimens should be cut with a large knife into thin slices, sparing the skin (Fig. 1-1). This is done by placing the breast specimen upside down on a plate. We place paper towels between the slices, which improves the penetration of the fixative. Then the specimen is immersed in a large volume of formalin. The mammilla should be cut off and fixed separately. The axillary content is fixed without previous incisions. Tumors and other pathologic lesions are carefully registered and measured before fixation. After fixation, we cut the axillary fat into thin slices. Every slice is then carefully palpated against a hard plate to find the lymph nodes, which are then picked out separately for histologic examination. The lymph nodes are sliced in 1-2-mm-thick slices, which are all embedded. The nodes are numbered either from the top or from the base of the axilla.

Various techniques have been advocated for the examination of the axillary lymph nodes, such as clearing of the specimens with xylene, serial sectioning or manual palpation of fresh or fixed specimens. We agree with Fisher and Slack (1970) that diligence in the search for metastases is more important than choice of technique. We have found the method recommended here to be accurate, simple and time-saving. With this method we have been able to find even more nodes than can be identified on radiographs of the specimens.

Samples covering at least one full cross-section of the tumor should be taken for histology, besides several additional samples from the central and marginal parts, depending on the size of the tumor. All breast tissue is again inspected macroscopically and blocks are taken from areas showing pathologic changes, as well from areas which appear grossly normal. No general rule can be given as to how many blocks should be taken from the grossly normal breast tissue. Since many precancerous and in situ lesions are not visible to the naked eye, the chance of diagnosing such lesions depends greatly on the extent of the histologic examination. At least 10-15 blocks from the non-tumorous parts of the breast are recommended in many current breast treatment programs. Many such programs also require the pathologist to take samples specifically from the four quadrants of the breast. Due to the loose consistency of breast tissue, allowing lesions to be pushed over wide areas, such attempts to localize lesions by the four quadrants provide a kind of false accuracy. A rough subdivision of the breast into a medial and a lateral half seems

more relevant practically speaking. The nipple is sliced according to Fig. 1-2.

The loose texture of breast tissue may also cause problems in deciding whether or not a lesion has been radically removed. The width of the margins is highly dependent on mechanical factors and radicality may sometimes be better evaluated macroscopically than on histologic sections from the marginal tissue, which may be highly deformed by the histologic processing.

Hematoxylin-eosin is suitable as a routine stain. Elastin stain and PAS-Alcian blue are also valuable in cases of carcinomas to evaluate elastin deposits in the stroma and mucinous substances in the tumor cells. We use these stains in all cases.

Formerly, frozen sections during operation were used in practically all cases of breast cancers and tumors suspected to be malignant. Due to the increasing accuracy of the preoperative diagnostic methods, mainly fine needle aspiration biopsy and mammography, the need for frozen section diagnostics has diminished. Today this procedure is rarely used, mostly in cases where the preoperative diagnostic parameters have not been in agreement. But even then, we tend to avoid this diagnostic measure.

Diagnosing on the basis of frozen sections is unreliable in lesions in an early stage of development, which (mainly due to health screening projects with mammography) constitute an increasing proportion of all surgical breast specimens. Precancerous lesions such as atypical epitheliosis and in situ carcinomas (intraductal and lobular) should not be diagnosed on frozen sections because of the high risk of misinterpretation. Paraffin sections of well fixed specimens are needed for a safe evaluation of such changes. Even infiltrating carcinomas, such as the lobular variant, growing diffusely in an otherwise preserved glandular tissue, may be very difficult to recognize on frozen sections. A further argument for reducing the number of frozen section examinations concerns the size of the lesion. Since the final histological diagnosis must be based on paraffin sections of unfrozen, well fixed specimens, the lesion may simply be too small to allow frozen sections to be cut as well. This situation is increasingly encountered, especially when tissue samples for steroid-receptor and DNA analyses are also required. It may also be useful in many cases to take samples for electron microscopy.

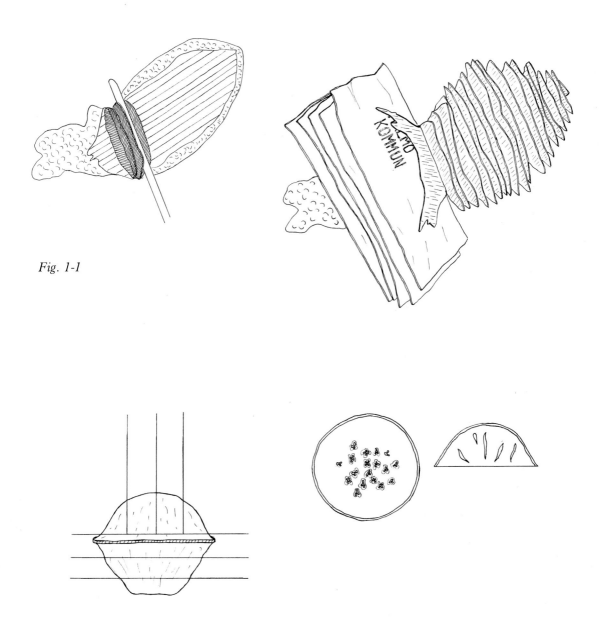

Fig. 1-1

Fig. 1-2

*Chapter 2*

# Normal Anatomy

## Histologic structure

Histologically the breast may be regarded as a compound alveolar ductal gland, each entity terminating in a lactiferous duct at the nipple. Before puberty the breast consists of a rather well demarcated mass of fibrous tissue with small ducts, lined by a single row of cuboidal epithelial cells, resting on a row of flat myothelial cells and surrounded by loose periductal stroma. At puberty, as a result of hormonal influences, a marked enlargement takes place from a development of the ductal system, formation of lobules and increase in the amount of stroma. This process continues beyond puberty, till about 30 years of age, when the female breast reaches the highest degree of structural and physiological development, surpassed only by the process of gestation.

Ch. 11 illustrates some histologic features of the normal adult female breast. *The mammillary collecting ducts* are illustrated in Fig. 11-1. Except for the most proximal part of the mammillary collecting ducts, which is lined by squamous epithelium, the ductal system and the lobular acini have principally the same epithelial set-up, i.e. a two-cell type structure consisting of a row of cuboidal or cylindrical epithelial cells resting on a row of myothelial cells. This distinctive feature of the normal structures is frequently preserved in various benign breast lesions, but deranged in most malignant processes. It may therefore serve as an important diagnostic criterion in the distinction between these two pathological conditions.

The *myothelium* may vary considerably in appearance, as shown in Figs. 11 – 2-4, and may undergo marked proliferative changes, also seen in various benign breast lesions such as sclerosing adenosis and papillomas (see Ch. 14).

The rare *clear cell lobules* are depicted in Fig. 11 – 5.

The various appearances of the *ducts* are illustrated in Fig. 11 – 6-7. The ducts are surrounded by a mantle of specialized stroma, which, in contrast to that of the lobules, also contains elastic fibers. This difference in the stromal component may persist under pathologic conditions and may be helpful in assessing the histogenetic relationships of various lesions. The amount of periductal elastin tends to increase with age and degree of parity. It also increases during various inflammatory processes affecting the ducts, a feature which may be relevant when discussing the pathogenesis of radial scars and the development of tubular carcinoma (see Ch. 14).

## Functional activity and cyclical changes

The lobular as well as the ductal systems are capable of secretion and absorption. Evidence of milk secretion may even be found in the normal breast during non-lactational periods in the form of *secretory lobules*, as illustrated in Fig. 11 – 8. But even apparently resting lobules and ducts produce small amounts of secretory products, e.g. various mucosubstances and fluid which are partly re-absorbed and partly transported to the surface via the ductal system. Blockage of ducts causes dilatation of the parts distal to the blockage, giving rise to retention mastitis (see Ch. 12). Apocrine tension cysts, which are a main feature in cystic breast disease (mastopathia cystica), develop because the absorptive processes cannot keep pace with the secretion of fluid by the apocrine epithelium. Since the outlet of such cysts is often blocked, the fluid accumulates under pressure.

Like the fallopian tube, cervix and vagina the breast tissue undergoes histologic variations which are associated with the *menstrual phase* and are due to the responsiveness of the breast tissue to the sexual hormones. These structural variations are briefly mentioned in Figs. 11 – 9-10 but we have refrained from giving detailed descriptions.

A marked proliferation of breast tissue may occur during *aldactone treatment*, as shown in Fig. 11 – 11.

The profound proliferative and secretory alterations which occur during *pregnancy* and *lactation* are shown in Figs. 11 – 12-15.

In Fig. 11 – 16 a case of *macromastia developing during pregnancy* is illustrated.

## Involution

Involution occurs after pregnancy and lactation and at the time of the menopause. Mammographic studies in recent years have contributed a great deal to our knowledge about this process but most of our information still concerns those changes which take place around the time of the menopause. Various examples of the *menopausal involution* are illustrated in Figs. 11 – 17-20.

All components of the glandular apparatus are involved. Also the interlobular supporting connective tissue is changed and to a varying degree replaced by adipose tissue, a process whose pathogenesis is still an enigma. The result of this alteration can be excellently visualized by mammography. The breasts from older women are usually far less electron dense than those of women in their fertile age period. This phenomenon is of great diagnostic importance since pathological processes, especially carcinomas, are easier to detect on mammograms from this age period. It is also important to bear this in mind when making statistical comparisons, for instance of the incidence of carcinoma between the two age groups.

During involution lobules may completely disappear, being replaced by fatty tissue. But sometimes only the tubules disappear, while the intralobular stroma becomes denser and may be converted into a dense hyaline mass. Such hyaline vestiges of lobules may merge with preexisting interlobular connective tissue, giving a false impression of fibrosis (Fig. 11 – 21). The adipose metaplasia proceeds unevenly in the breast, which may result in a granular or even nodular consistency on palpation. Sometimes the adipose metaplasia may even isolate a larger area of persisting fibrous stroma, which may produce an impression of a tumor by palpation or mammographically, resulting in surgical excision. It is natural, then, that the pathologist who examines such a specimen may be tempted to make the diagnosis of *"fibrosis"*. The pathologic diagnosis "fibrosis mammae" more often illustrates the pathologist's desire to satisfy the surgeon's need for a justification of surgical intervention than it represents a designation of a true pathologic process.

In the duct system similar epithelial changes occur as in the lobules, but whether, or to what extent, there is also an actual disappearance of ducts is not known. In breasts from older women we have sometimes seen a marked hyaline sclerosis around ducts with atrophic epithelium but we do not know whether these changes are sequelae of previous inflammation or represent true, physiologic involution. Interestingly, we have observed similar changes of ducts, involved by intraductal carcinoma (see Ch. 15). In such instances, however, we have often also found varying degrees of round cell infiltration around such ducts, indicating that an inflammatory component has been involved in these particular cases. Likewise, we are not sure whether the increase in elastin around larger ducts which occurs with increasing age is purely involutionary or pathologic.

A special form of involution resulting in a picture reminiscent of gynecomastia may occur in *anorexia nervosa,* as is shown in Fig. 11 – 22.

In Fig. 11 – 23 we illustrate *fibrosis after radiation.*

# Chapter 3

# Inflammatory Changes

The anatomical structure of the breast, containing a ductal system which connects the glandular apparatus with the skin surface creates possibilities for an invasion of pathogenic microorganisms into the breast.

Figs. 12 – 1-2 deal with various forms of *unspecific mastitis*. Infective granulomas, such as tuberculosis, syphilis, lepra and rare mycotic infections are not considered in this book, since they show no special features in the breast.

The peculiar condition called *"granulomatous mastitis"*, which should be distinguished from tuberculous mastitis, is illustrated in Fig. 12 – 3.

*Sarcoid reactions* in association with carcinoma of the breast are described in Fig. 12 – 4.

The various stages of the common condition called the *"retention syndrome"*, including duct-

ectasia, retention mastitis and obliterative mastopathy, and the controversial term *"plasma cell mastitis"* are discussed in Figs. 12 – 5-9.

*Necrosis of the breast* is not especially illustrated. Most cases of breast necrosis are traumatic. Extensive hemorrhagic necrosis may develop following anticoagulant therapy with coumarin and indanedione derivatives. This complication, which is very rare, results in a total or subtotal ischemic infarction of the breast. Venous thrombosis of the neck may occasionally also be associated with ischemic infarction.

Tissue reaction patterns to various forms of *breast prosthesis* such as ivalon and silicone prostheses are discussed in Figs. 12 – 10-11.

*Chapter 4*

# Benign Tumors and Tumor-like Lesions

Fibroadenoma is the most common benign tumor of the breast. These tumors characteristically develop during the fertile period as circumscribed and mostly solitary growths which have a characteristic microscopic structure.

*Fibroadenomas* are illustrated in Figs. 13 – 1-5. The stroma of fibroadenomas may show structural variability according to the age of the patient, a phenomenon which, in turn, is probably related to the hormonal background. A pronounced *myxomatous stroma* is often seen in tumors removed from young women, as seen in Fig. 13 – 3. This feature is also conspicuous in *juvenile fibroadenoma* which may reach a large size (giant fibroadenoma) and is illustrated in Fig. 13 – 4. Likewise, during pregnancy and lactation fibroadenomas may undergo an accelerated growth with proliferation of ducts and formation of lobular acini showing evidence of secretion and lactation.

After lactation and menopause fibroadenomas undergo involutionary changes very similar to those seen in normal breast tissue. A tumor removed from an old woman showing an unusual *elastosis* of the stroma is shown in Fig. 13 – 5.

Various manifestations of cystic disease (see Ch. 5), quite frequent findings in non-tumorous breast tissue, may also develop in fibroadenomas. Thus *apocrine metaplasia* as well as

*epitheliosis* may be found in these tumors, as seen in Fig. 13 – 6 and 13 – 7, respectively. Azzopardi has described a peculiar form of epitheliosis showing a proliferation of clear, argyrophil cells of *"endocrine type"* within the tubules and ducts of the tumor. This phenomenon has been claimed to represent an endocrine differentiation of the duct epithelium. Whether it is truly endocrine, however, remains to be proven.

Fibroadenomas, like normal lobules and ducts, may be involved in *lobular carcinoma in situ* as well as in *intraductal carcinoma of comedo type*. These are discussed in Figs. 13 – 8 and 13 – 9, respectively.

*Pure adenoma* and *lactating adenoma* are entities whose relationship to fibroadenomas and hamartomas is controversial. These problems are discussed in Fig. 13 – 10.

*Hamartomas* and their various histologic appearances are illustrated in Figs. 13 – 11-14.

*Intraductal papilloma*, so-called *papillomatosis* and *juvenile papillomatosis* are discussed in Figs. 13 – 15-18. *"Swiss-cheese disease"* is a rather vaguely defined designation which may represent variants of juvenile papillomatosis, although some cases, reported under this name, undoubtedly are examples of cystic breast disease. This item is discussed further in Figs. 13 – 19-20.

*Chapter 5*

# Cystic Breast Disease and Related Conditions Precancerous Lesions

"Cystic breast disease" and "cystic mastopathy" are probably the most commonly used names for clinically as well as pathologically rather ill-defined and poorly understood conditions. Although it is commonly believed that the underlying cause of these changes is related to an abnormality in the responsiveness of the glandular tissue to hormonal (preferably estrogen) stimuli, our knowledge of the exact nature of the condition is rather meager. Furthermore, its demarcation from normal, physiological changes such as proliferation and involution is not clearly defined. This has caused a great deal of vagueness in the diagnosis of cystic disease, which has come to include a wide range of different histologic changes. Traditionally, cystic breast disease has been understood to include macro- and microcysts, glandular hyperplasias such as sclerosing adenosis and "blunt duct adenosis", ductal hyperplasias and epitheliosis as well as apocrine change of the epithelium. But sometimes fibrosis, fibroadenoma and papilloma are also included under this heading. Our ignorance of the true nature of the condition is well illustrated by the number of more or less unsuitable names proposed for it, such as mastopathy, mammary dysplasia, fibroadenosis, chronic mastitis and cystic mastitis, although, admittedly, most of these names have

now been abandoned by most pathologists. We believe that cystic disease is due to an alteration in the relation between hormonal influence and end organ tissue response, and that there certainly exist extremes and the distinction between normal and pathological is diffuse. It may well be that the diversity of "lesions" usually included in the term "cystic disease" merely represents a spectrum of changes, all of which have been induced by a common causal principle and that some forms (e.g. the microscopic form so often seen incidentally in breast specimens and without clinical significance) may be looked upon as variants of normal conditions. These ideas have been excellently discussed by Love et al. (1982) to whom we refer for further reading.

Various histologic changes found in *cystic disease* are illustrated in Figs. 14 – 1-3.

The *"benign calcifications"* seen in mammographic pictures are often present in connection with lobular involution and cystic disease but may also occur in old hyalinized fibroadenomas (Figs. 14 – 4-5). However, mammographic calcifications may also be an indication of carcinoma. Some, but not all, *"malignant calcifications"* have a distinctive appearance, viz. those occurring in intraductal carcinoma of comedo type (Fig. 14 – 6).

Various forms of *adenosis* are discussed in Ch. 14. *Sclerosing adenosis* is illustrated in Figs. 14 – 7-10. A special variant, called *"intraductal sclerosing adenosis"*, showing intraductal proliferations, is discussed in Figs. 14 – 11-12.

A curious *"ducto-tubular" form* of sclerosing adenosis is shown in Fig. 14 – 13.

*"Adenosis tumor"* is a lesion which we believe is closely related to sclerosing adenosis, being a tumor-like form of this condition. It is an important lesion since it may, clinically and histopathologically, be mistaken for a malignant tumor. An example of this lesion is illustrated in Fig. 14 – 14.

*Microglandular adenosis*, as defined by McDivitt et al. (1968) is discussed in Figs. 14 – 15-17. The nature of this lesion and its possible relationship to sclerosing adenosis is enigmatic. It appears to be a benign process which should be distinguished from tubular carcinoma. Recently, several papers about this poorly understood condition have appeared (see references).

*Epitheliosis* is understood here as a benign solid papillary or cribriform epithelial proliferation within ducts, tubules and/or lobules. It is a common component of cystic disease but may also occur without this association. It has been claimed that cystic disease carries an increased risk for the development into carcinoma, although this has been difficult to prove statistically (see Love et al., 1982). It has been suspected that the component of epitheliosis in cystic disease could be the structural basis for such a malignant change. On the other hand, it has also been propounded that intraductal carcinoma more often may arise *de novo* from normal cells passing through a phase of atypical hyperplasia, which is distinct from the epitheliosis occurring as a component of cystic disease (see Azzopardi, 1979). This, however, would be difficult to prove in practice. In Figs. 14 – 18-23 we discuss several examples of

epitheliosis with varying degrees of cytologic atypia and frank intraductal carcinoma, sometimes coexisting and thus suggesting a gradual transition from benign hyperplasia to carcinoma.

A special form of epitheliosis, called *"cribriform lobular atypia"* and its relationship to lobular carcinoma in situ is discussed in Figs. 14 – 24-25.

Under the name of *"radial scar"* we understand a special type of sclerotic lesion which in earlier days did not arouse any special interest but which has proved to be very common and important in cancerogenesis. Radial scars have been described under various names:
– "Rosette-like lesions; proliferation centres" (Semb, 1928),
– "sclerosing papillary proliferations" (Fenoglio & Lattes, 1974),
– "strahlige Narben" (Hamperl, 1975),
– "benign sclerosing ductal proliferation" (Tremblay et al., 1977),
– "nonencapsulated sclerosing lesions" (Fisher et al., 1979),
– "infiltrating epitheliosis" (Azzopardi, 1979), and
– "radial scars" = translation of the term used by Hamperl (Linell et al. 1980).

As early as 1928 Semb thought they were starting points for carcinoma. Their benign nature has been emphasized by Fenoglio & Lattes. Fisher et al. stated that "these lesions may represent incipient tubular carcinoma". Our studies have convinced us that radial scars are the starting points for tubular carcinomas.

For a full discussion of the literature on radial scar we refer to Linell et al. (1980).

The occurrence and morphology of *radial scars* are described in Figs. 14 – 26-49. In this section there are also descriptions of the *development of tubular carcinoma in radial scars*. The pathogenesis of radial scars is also discussed and in this connection the *terminal ductolobular unit* of Wellings-Jensen and its relation to cancerogenesis is treated (see especially Figs. 14 – 42-43. In the development of radial scars *obliterative lesions* in ducts probably play an important role (Figs. 14 – 45-49 and Fig. 15 – 43.

The terminal ductolobular unit of Wellings-Jensen has been especially emphasized by them in the pathogenesis of ductal carcinomas of comedo-type and their pictures show outfolded lobules with epithelial proliferations. The radial scars are probably situated in the same region of the branching breast glands as the terminal duc-tolobular unit. Then it is not astonishing to find development of both comedo carcinomas and lobular carcinomas in close connection to radial scars. We have repeatedly observed changes of this type and we will illustrate them in the section on combined carcinomas in Ch. 15-82-87. The limited space does not allow to illustrate these questions more extensively. Even if there is a close connection between different types of breast carcinomas, these combined types are a relatively small proportion of breast carcinomas.

# Chapter 6

# Carcinomas

## Current classifications

Over the years a large number of classifications, more or less elaborated, have been proposed for breast carcinoma. Many of them are merely modifications of earlier classifications. In recent years the most widely used classification has been the one proposed by Fisher et al. (1975). Their classification for invasive carcinomas is given below.

1. *Infiltrating ductal* without special features or not otherwise specified (NOS type).
2. Medullary.
3. Lobular invasive.
4. Mucinous.
5. Tubular.
6. Adenocystic.
7. Papillary.
8. Carcinosarcoma.
9. Paget's disease.
10. Combinations with NOS type (25-30% of carcinomas).
11. Combinations without NOS type (rare cases).

The last edition of WHO "Histological typing of breast tumours" has a more elaborated classification of malignant epithelial tumors.

1. Noninvasive.
   a. intraductal carcinoma
   b. lobular carcinoma in situ.
2. Invasive.
   a. invasive ductal carcinoma
   b. invasive ductal carcinoma with a predominant intraductal component
   c. invasive lobular carcinoma
   d. mucinous carcinoma
   e. medullary carcinoma
   f. papillary carcinoma
   g. tubular carcinoma
   h. adenoid-cystic carcinoma
   i. secretory (juvenile) carcinoma
   j. apocrine carcinoma
   k. carcinoma with metaplasia
   l. others.
3. Paget's disease of the nipple.

In both of these classifications ductal carcinomas NOS or invasive ductal carcinomas constitute the majority of carcinomas, whereas the tubular variety is very rare (1-2%).

## Histogenetic aspects

From the foregoing chapter we have propounded the theory that a large number of carcinomas (tubular) start in radial scars. In screening materials of breast carcinoma tubular carcinoma may constitute a considerable part (> 20%). During our studies we have, on purely histologic grounds, arrived at the conclusion that a large part (about 50% in our material) of breast carcinomas have developed by tumor progression from tubular carcinomas originating in radial scars.

For a deeper discussion with all arguments we must refer to our book from 1980 (Linell et al.).

It was already known earlier that tubular carcinoma is seldom purely tubular but contains an admixture of less differentiated "ductal" structures. This term "ductal" in quotation marks may seem difficult to understand and meaningless. Nevertheless, we have used it here because it is so widespread. It is, however, understandable only when considering the terminology from a historical point of view. From the beginning the common view was held that carcinomas start from ductal epithelium and should therefore be called ductal carcinomas, and they were divided into scirrhous and medullary (encephaloid) variants. Later, some special carcinomas were distinguished. Lobular carcinomas were well known after Foote & Stewart's work in the forties and were called "lobular" because the in situ form appeared to originate in lobules.

Other special forms were mucinous (colloid) carcinoma and medullary carcinoma with lymphoid stroma infiltration. Around 1970 tubular carcinoma (well differentiated adenocarcinoma) was separated as a distinct type, although it was described more than 100 years ago. All these special forms were looked upon as various examples of ductal carcinomas. After their separation, there remained a very large group (75-85% of all carcinomas) called "ductal carcinoma without special signs" (Saphir, 1958) or "ductal carcinoma NOS (not otherwise specified)" (Fisher et al., 1975). These classifications have often been ascribed to Foote & Stewart without realizing that Foote & Stewart in fact divided ductal carcinomas into those with progressive fibrosis and those called "comedo carcinoma". In these classifications the meaning of the term "ductal" has gradually changed, to be used in the sense of growing in columns and strands without any special structures as glandular or papillary formations. Nowadays "ductal" has lost even more of its meaning since there is increasing evidence that these carcinomas start in lobules (Fig. 15 – 43). Even the term "lobular" in the sense of a carcinoma starting in the lobules seems to be losing its identity. Changes in the ducts are practically always seen in lobular carcinoma and we cannot exclude the possibility that this tumor starts in ducts. Summarizing, there are indications that "ductal" and "lobular" have lost their original meaning in the histogenetic sense.

With adequate sampling of tubular carcinoma we could always find abundant elastin as remnants of radial scars. Through extensive histologic analysis such remnants could be traced in a large group of carcinomas which also could be placed in a series showing a decreasing amount of tubules and an increasing proportion of less differentiated "ductal" structures ending up with a tumor variety totally devoid of tubules and wholly made up of "ductal" structures. The carcinomas in this large group were further characterized by having moderate cellular atypia. Intraductal growth was less conspicuous and cancerization of lobules practically never seen.

On the basis of these properties we created a series of what we called tubuloductal carcinomas, which could semiquantitatively be divided into five sub-classes, as given below.

| 1. tubular carcinoma ++++ | = pure tubular carcinoma |
| 2. tubular carcinoma +++ | = preponderantly tubular with admixture of less differentiated "ductal" structures |
| 3. tubular carcinoma ++ | = tubules and "ductal" structures in roughly equal proportions |
| 4. tubular carcinoma + | = only a few tubules, mainly "ductal" structures |

5. tubular carcinoma 0 = no tubules, only "ductal" structures.

All these types were characterized by sclerotic centers with abundant elastin deposits. The cells were not very polymorphous. Intraductal growth (mostly cribriform but sometimes papillary or solid during progression) was occasionally seen. Outgrowth into the lobules ("cancerization of lobules") was practically never seen.

This idea of a serial progression of tubular carcinoma to less differentiated forms was originally a purely histologic concept. Statistical studies were therefore instigated, especially on the relation between tumor size and frequency of axillary lymph node metastases. The results from the years 1976-78 were published earlier (Linell et al., 1980). The material from two later periods have since been added and these results are shown in Table 6-1. It is obvious that the correlation found between tumor size and frequency of node metastases in the axilla, interpreted as strong support for our progression theory, has been further substantiated with the larger material.

In our earlier book we used other arguments (the nature of metastases, the mammographic picture), which further supported the progression theory, as the most probable explanation for the development of tubuloductal carcinoma. In later years the DNA-profiles of tumors have been studied (Pontén et al.). Tumors included in the groups tubular carcinoma ++++ or +++ were often found to be euploid whereas tubular carcinomas ++, + or 0 were mostly aneuploid, findings which are in accord with the concept of tumor progression as the most likely mechanism by which the tubuloductal carcinomas evolve.

As previously described common classifications from later years usually include a very large group (constituting 75-85%) called "ductal carcinoma", often with the adding of NOS (not otherwise specified). From this large group our "tubuloductal carcinomas" (about 50% in our material) were collected. The remaining fraction consists of a group of tumors (about 20% in our material) which we have called "ductal carcinoma of comedo type".

On the basis of our studies we have proposed a classification which can be regarded as a modification of earlier classifications.

*Table 6-1. Tubular and tubuloductal cancer 1976-78, 1976-80 and 1976-81.*

| Tubular carcinoma | No. of Cases | | | Mean diam. (cm) | | | % axillary metastases | | |
|---|---|---|---|---|---|---|---|---|---|
| | 1976-78 | 1976-80 | 1976-81 | 1976-78 | 1976-80 | 1976-81 | 1976-78 | 1976-80 | 1976-81 |
| ++++ | 39 | 64 | 73 | 0.8 | 0.8 | 0.9 | 11 | 17 | 16 |
| +++ | 56 | 81 | 94 | 1.4 | 1.3 | 1.5 | 31 | 30 | 29 |
| ++ | 50 | 98 | 117 | 1.7 | 1.5 | 1.5 | 36 | 37 | 36 |
| + | 70 | 109 | 134 | 2.0 | 1.9 | 1.9 | 51 | 49 | 47 |
| 0 | 47 | 59 | 66 | 2.5 | 2.7 | 2.3 | 52 | 58 | 50 |

## Proposed classification

I. *Carcinoma in situ*

A. Lobular carcinoma in situ (Lcis or Clis)
B. Intraductal carcinoma ("comedo" type) including Paget's nipple disease.

II. *Invasive carcinoma*

| *Invasive* | *Precancerous or in situ lesion* |
|---|---|
| A. Invasive lobular carcinoma. | Lobular carcinoma in situ? |
| B. Tubular* and tubuloductal carcinoma. | Radial scar. |
| C. Ductal carcinoma of "comedo" type. | Intraductal carcinoma (solid, papillary, cribriform, or mural). |
| D. Medullary carcinoma with lymphoid infiltration | Probably intraductal carcinoma. |
| E. Mucinous (colloid) carcinoma. | Probably intraductal carcinoma. |
| F. Rare types of breast carcinoma. | Not known. |
|     a. Adenoid-cystic carcinoma. | |
|     b. Secretory (infantile). | |
|     c. Lipid-rich. | |
|     d. Carcinoid. | |
|     e. Metaplastic. | |
|     f. Nipple carcinoma. | Probably florid adenomatosis of the nipple. |

* We include in tubular carcinoma the "invasive cribriform carcinoma", published by Page et al. (1983).

## Frequencies of different carcinomas

We do not give any frequency figures because these vary a great deal in different materials unless they are very carefully defined to permit comparison. Old materials composed of rather large tumors, diagnosed only by palpation, differ greatly from materials derived from mammographic screening projects. Likewise there are differences between materials derived from the first, the second, etc., screening as well as materials of carcinomas diagnosed between screenings ("interval carcinomas") (Sigfusson & Andersson). Age distribution may also influence the frequency of different types of carcinoma.

## Comparison with other classifications

The only real difference between our classification and other current classifications is that the latter separate tubular carcinoma as a distinct and special type, while we incorporate tubular carcinoma as one stage in a series of common carcinomas showing varying degrees of progression from the most differentiated pure tubular carcinoma to less differentiated types. Our five types, created for scientific studies, may look impractical. We have therefore, in daily practice proposed lumping tubular carcinoma ++++ and tubular carcinoma +++ together as tubular carcinoma and use the term "tubuloductal carcinoma" for tubular carcinoma ++, tubular carcinoma + and tubular carcinoma 0.

Otherwise the carcinoma groups proposed by us are to be found in many other classifications. Foote & Stewart did not know of tubular carcinomas, but they divided "ductal" carcinomas into ductal carcinoma with progressive fibrosis and comedo carcinoma. This subdivision corresponds closely to Azzopardi's stellate or irregular ductal carcinoma and multinodular, knobby or circumscribed ductal carcinoma.

Inspired by our classification Fisher et al. (1983) in a comprehensive study of 1600 cases divide the ductal carcinomas into two groups: a) scar carcinomas (including tubular carcinoma) and b) non-scar carcinomas. There are differences in interpretation but on the whole there seems to be a very good agreement between their grouping and our groups of tubuloductal and comedo carcinoma. Scar cancer constituted 38% in their material, which is rather old, consisting of many large tumors.

WHO (1981) follows the proposition of Saphir (1958) and Fisher et al. (1975) and lumps these two types together as invasive ductal carcinoma. WHO has a special group called "invasive ductal carcinoma with a predominant intraductal component". The separation of such a group may be practical but is not logically motivated.

Most classifications list papillary carcinomas as a special group. We have never seen a pure papillary carcinoma and regard this variety as belonging to comedo carcinoma. It may be justified to use the description papillary carcinoma when papillary structures are a very prominent feature.

For further studies on problems of classification, the references to Ch. 6 and Ch. 15 may be consulted.

## Prognostic implications of classification

Over the years a large number of studies have been performed to try to correlate histologic type and prognosis. A statistic correlation has sometimes been found but the success has mostly been meager. In the classifications used in these studies the vast majority of cases will be placed in *one* large group (i.e. ductal carcinoma NOS). Therefore it can a priori be said that such histologic classifications will be of very little value in predicting the course.

We have of course been interested in these questions to see whether our classification offers advantages from a prognostic point of view. We can only relate a few pilot studies; these, however, appear promising. In this connection we would like to refer to the results achieved so far from a study of a part of our large material, which has been reclassified by one of us (F.L.). This material (see Borgström & Linell) comprises those cases during 1969-75 classified clinically as being in stage 1 (= without axillary metastases). In this material, as in others of this type, the clinical classification was found to be wrong in about 30% of the cases. The cases had been randomized, half of the patients having been treated by simple mastectomy and the other half also with axillary *exeresis*. As the mortality was the same in both groups we have lumped them together, giving 188 cases in all. They have been followed for 8-14 years. Practically all the patients who died were autopsied. The results are given in Table 6-2.

The small groups are without interest in this rather small material; we concentrated on the two groups "Tubuloductal cancer" and "Inva-

Table 6-2.

| | No. cases | Dead No. | % | Dead with cancer at autopsy No. | % |
|---|---|---|---|---|---|
| Intraductal comedo cancer | 21 | 0 | 0 | 0 | 0 |
| Invasive comedo cancer | 50 | 19 | 38 | 17 | 34 |
| Tubular cancer ++++ | 11 } 24 | 2 | 8 | 0 | 0 |
| Tubular cancer +++ | 13 | | | | |
| Tubular cancer ++ | 23 } 74 | 9 | 12 | 7 | 10 |
| Tubular cancer + | 16 } 50 | 7 | 14 | 7 | 14 |
| Tubular cancer 0 | 11 | | | | |
| Medullary cancer with lymphoid stroma infiltration | 22 | 9 | 41 | 3 | 14 |
| Lobular carcinoma | 17 | 7 | 41 | 5 | 29 |
| Mucinous cancer | 3 | 0 | 0 | 0 | 0 |
| Adenoid cystic cancer | 1 | 0 | 0 | 0 | 0 |
| | 188 | 44 | 23 | 39 | 21 |

sive comedo cancer". The differences in mortality are obvious and may point to a fundamental biological difference between these two groups. This indicates that our classification may have a high predictive value, although further studies are needed.

This book is especially intended to arouse interest in our classification with the hope that it will be used on different materials. In this way it may be possible to gain knowledge about its prognostic value as compared with staging, grading, DNA-studies of ploidi, assessment of hormone receptors and other, more or less sophisticated, parameters.

## Description of the atlas part

Many of the problems discussed here are treated in more detail in the atlas part of this book. The development of *tubular carcinoma* and its histologic properties are to be found in Figs. 14 – 26-48 and Figs. 15 – 1-12. *Tubuloductal carcinoma* (Invasive ductal carcinoma) is described in Figs. 15 – 13-27 and *comedo carcinoma* of different types in Figs. 15 – 28-45. The closely related *mucinous carcinoma* and *medullary carcinoma with lymphoid infiltration* are treated in Figs. 15 – 46-54. *Lobular carcinoma* (in situ and invasive) is illustrated in Figs. 15 – 55-71. Several *special* and *rare types* are to be found in Figs. 15 – 72-81. Under this heading we have listed some types which are distinctive and others which are probably variants of the main forms.

In the first category we count *adenoid-cystic carcinoma*, Fig. 15 – 72-74, *secretory (infantile) carcinoma*, Fig. 15 – 75, and *metaplastic carcinoma*, Fig. 15 – 79. In the other group we put *carcinoma with giant cells*, Fig. 15 – 78, *lipid rich carcinoma*, Figs. 15 – 76-77, and *breast carcinoma with argyrophil cells – carcinoid tumor?* (Figs. 15 – 80-81).

In Figs. 15 – 82-84 the important problem of *combined types of carcinoma* in one tumor is considered. When using a classification with the large group ductal carcinoma NOS (not otherwise specified) this problem will be concealed, but using our classification combined carcinoma types will emerge sooner or later.

Fig. 15 – 85 discusses, in connection with a case, the important question of *bilateral carcinoma*.

In Figs. 15 – 86-87 an interesting case of *multiple carcinomas in monozygote twins* is described, resulting in considerations about *occult* and *hereditary conditioned carcinoma*.

*Regression of carcinoma* in the breast as in many other places is a very controversial theme. That we really can have regression of malignant tumors seems to be beyond any doubt in the case of malignant melanoma and renal carcinoma. In the breast pictures are sometimes seen suggesting a spontaneous destruction of the carcinoma. This is especially found in *intraductal comedo carcinoma*. Figs. 15 – 88-91 contain pictures of this type. The dilemma is always that we cannot be assured that it is a regressed carcinoma unless we have some remnants of vital tumor and then we cannot be certain that the regression will be total. Figs. 15 – 92-93 describe a case of *tubuloductal carcinoma* with structures which we hypothetically have interpreted as signs of *regression*. Figs. 15 – 53-54 show widespread *spontaneous necroses in medullary carcinoma with lymphoid stroma infiltration*. Those can also be interpreted as signs of regression, possibly on an immunologic basis.

Extensive histologic studies of breast specimens (Ringberg, Palmer & Linell, 1982 with references) have revealed the frequent occurrence of multiple and contralateral carcinomas. Studies of the frequency of clinically manifest carcinomas support the hypothesis that many carcinomas remain quiescent or even regress.

*Lymph node metastases* from different kinds of carcinoma are illustrated in Figs. 15 – 10-11, 15 – 15, 15 – 54 and 15 – 60.

In this chapter we illustrate some *atypical metastases*. Figs. 15 – 94-96 (from comedo carcinoma, tubuloductal and lobular carcinoma) show metastatic growth that resembles *intraductal growth*. Obviously this cannot be the truth, the pictures in fact illustrate tumor growth in lymph vessels. This raises questions about the interpretation of intraductal growth in the breast, often taken as proof of primary growth. In most cases this probably does represent growth in ducts of the breast, but it is essential to be cautious in the interpretations of lesions of this type.

Fig. 15 – 97 shows *unusual elastin production* in a metastasis of a tubuloductal carcinoma reminiscent of the elastin deposits seen in radial scars and tubular carcinomas (see Ch. 14 and Ch. 15).

# Chapter 7

# Mesenchymal Tumors

Most cases of this group are not characteristic for the breast tissue but are to be regarded as soft tissue tumors which happen to develop in the breast.

The only specific breast tumor among them is "*cystosarcoma phyllodes*". This very controversial tumor, consisting of both stromal and epithelial elements, is considered in Figs. 16 – 1-10. They mostly behave in a benign fashion, although the course in the individual case is usually unpredictable. When malignant change occurs this mostly involves the stromal component. Pure *mesenchymal tumors* (liposarcoma, myosarcoma, fibrosarcoma, chondrosarcoma, and osteosarcoma) are rarely encountered in the breast. Since they have the same properties as in other locations we will only discuss a few examples of this category (Figs. 16 – 11-12) just to remind the reader of their existence. For more detailed information we refer to books on soft tissue tumors.

A special mention is given to *angioma* (Fig. 16 – 13, and *angiosarcoma* (Fig. 16 – 14-15), because these tumors are the ones seen most often. But *angiosarcomas* (lymph- and hemangiosarcomas), developing in *lymphoedematous tissue (Stewart-Treves syndrome)*, mostly in the extremities, are not discussed. Their only connection with the breast lies in the fact that they are most frequent in the lymphoedematous arms after mastectomies with removal of axillary tissue.

*Chapter 8*

# Mammillary Diseases

From a practical point of view we have collected diseases of the nipple in a separate chapter. Some of these diseases are not specific for the nipple, but features reflecting diseases in other parts of the breast.

Other diseases may be found in the skin in other places of the body but have a predilection for the nipple.

Fig. 17 – 1 treats *Paget's disease,* which is a carcinomatous invasion of the epidermis. Controversial opinions are presented. Nowadays it seems quite clear that it is an intraductal carcinoma of comedo type secondarily invading the epidermis. It appears to be essential that the carcinoma cells reach the epidermis via the milk ducts, since Paget's disease is never found when a carcinoma reaches the epidermis outside the areola. It is also essential that it is an intraductal carcinoma of comedo type. *Other types of carcinoma* (see Fig. 17 – 2) do not cause Paget's disease, which seems to point to a profound biologic difference between comedo carcinoma and other breast carcinomas. It is interesting that an extra-mammillary Paget's disease also exists mostly in the axillae or in the perineal region. In at least 50% of the cases of extra-mammillary Paget's disease an underlying carcinoma in apocrine sweat glands is found. We do not know if the remaining 50% of cases develop primarily in the epidermis or if an underlying carcinoma has been overlooked due to inadequate sampling. It has been claimed that a small proportion of cases (up to 20%) of Paget's nipple disease are not associated with a concomitant comedo carcinoma. Toker has suggested a possible origin for these cases in "clear cells" in the epidermis of the nipple.

*Paget's disease* is rather rare (1-2% in most materials of breast cancer). It may be confined to the nipple, but frequently, it is part of a widespread comedo cancer in the breast. In such cases Paget's changes in the epithelium may develop without clinical symptoms.

An important lesion is *florid adenomatosis* or *adenoma of the nipple,* treated in Figs. 17 – 3-6. These tumors are usually benign but they may show *malignant potential* and may develop into *frank nipple carcinoma* Figs. 17 – 7-8).

The nipple is a predilection site for *lymphadenosis benigna cutis* (Bäfverstedt's disease or Spiegler Fendt's sarcoid), illustrated in Fig. 17 – 9.

*Parasites (Demodex folliculorum)* are often seen in the nipple without causing disease (Fig. 17 – 10).

*Chapter 9*

# Diseases of the Male Breast

*Gynecomastia.* This represents development of breast tissue under the nipple in males. In newborn male children there is a development of ducts due to estrogenic influence during intrauterine life. This regresses more or less completely. But after estrogen stimulation the breast tissue may again develop. Most cases are seen in adolescents, which are believed to be due to a reversible hormonal imbalance brought about by an increase in the pituitary gonadotropin and STH secretion during this age period. Gynecomastia can be uni- or bilateral. Unilateral cases may seem difficult to explain if the cause is a general hormonal disturbance, but could be due to differences in the amount of glandular tissue responsive to hormonal influences on the two sides.

Many cases of gynecomastia are due to hormone producing tumors or liver diseases with deficient breakdown of estrogens. The most common type of gynecomastia is iatrogenic and seen in patients with cancer of the prostate treated with estrogens. Andersen & Gram (1982) have made interesting studies on gynecomastia and have shown that this condition is much more common (about 50%) at autopsy than in clinical materials. They have also made plausible that gynecomastia is a disease with an early active phase and a late sclerotic, inactive phase (see Figs. 18 – 1-3).

*Carcinoma* in the male breast is rather rare, mostly with a frequency lower than 1%. The frequency is different in different countries and materials. In our material the frequency is close to 0,1%.

All types of carcinoma seen in the female breast are also seen in the male and therefore we have no illustrations but refer to the female breast carcinomas.

*Metastases* of carcinoma in the male breast are seen mostly in gynecomastia after treatment of prostatic cancer with estrogens. The metastases are mostly from the carcinoma of the prostate (Berge, 1971; Berge & Lundberg, 1977).

# Chapter 10

# Varia

In this chapter we have collected a few lesions which do not fit into any other chapter. Common to these changes is the fact that they are not specific for the breast but can be found in many other localities. Their main importance is in differential diagnosis.

Examples of *sweat gland tumors* are to be found in Figs. 19 – 1-5.

*Infiltrating fibromatosis* (Fig. 19 – 6-7) is of differential-diagnostic importance.

Some lesions and diseases appearing in the breast have not been handled in this book. In this respect we mentioned earlier a series of specific infections. In many textbooks *subcutaneous phlebitis* (Mondor's disease) is listed as a specific breast disease. This is wrong as it can be seen anywhere on the body (see references).

*Part Two*

# Color Atlas

*Chapter 11*

# Normal Anatomy

*Fig. 11-1*

*Normal mammilla.* The mammilla is the most prominent part of the breast and it seems appropriate that the atlas starts with this structure.

The pictures show the mammilla from a 60-year-old woman cut according to the principles put forward in Ch. 1. To the left a vertical section of the top. These 3 or 4 vertical sections show the skin (important for diagnosing Paget's disease, Ch. 15). We see only 4 ducts in this section. To the right, a section parallel to the skin surface a little lower in the mammilla. These sections are necessary to show all the ducts, 27 in this case. An intraductal carcinoma with Paget's disease is often confined to one or just a few ducts and would easily have been missed if only vertical sections had been made. The epithelium lining the milk ducts, which are often starshaped, is double-layered.

There can be up to 35-40 milk ducts or sinuses but most of them end blindly. In deeper sections of the mammilla the number is mostly reduced to 5-9. At the same level smaller ducts and lobules are seen to bud from the milk ducts. The larger milk ducts form the cores of the breast lobes, said to be 5-9 in number. As far as we know, no one has been able to dissect the breast lobes, which would be of utmost interest for the study of breast diseases.

*Fig. 11-2*

*Myothelium.* The following pictures illustrate the stratification of cells in ducts and lobules to show the normal variations in appearance. These variations are partly real, some are artifacts due to variation in fixation, etc.

To the left a couple of ducts from a 52-year-old woman. The epithelium is distinct from the myothelial cells. The latter are vacuolated, which may be a fixation artifact.

To the right a lobule where the myothelial cells are light eosinophil and attenuated for some length.

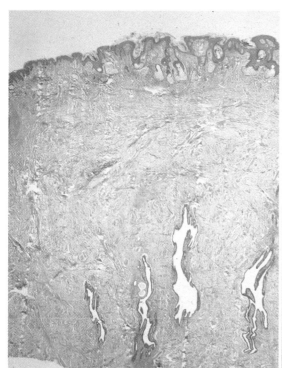

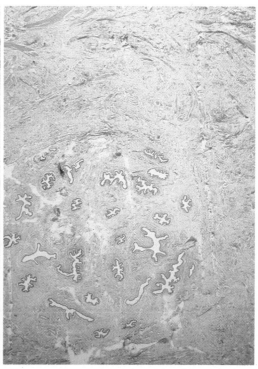

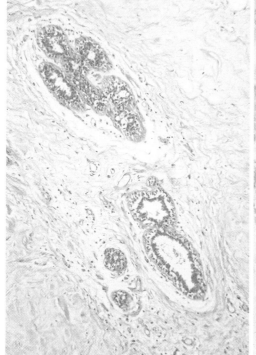

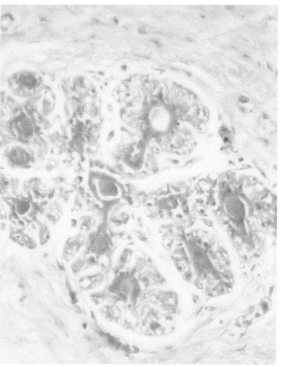

*Fig. 11-3*

*Myothelium.* Sometimes the myothelium is very pronounced and the ducts look like eosinophil strands of longish cells.

To the upper left, a part of a lobule from a 48-year-old woman. In the lower part, a lobule with a duct with very conspicuous eosinophil myothelium.

To the right, a detail of this duct. The picture may imitate epithelial growth in a nerve, a feature sometimes found in sclerosing adenosis. This pitfall was already pointed out by Davies (1973), who described epithelial growth in nerves in sclerosing adenosis (see Ch. 14).

*Fig. 11-4*

*Myothelial islands.* These structures have been especially described by Hamperl and are something inbetween normal tissue and sclerosing adenosis.

To the left, three small lobules from a 58-year-old woman. The lower one shows a special feature called a myoepithelial island. A conglomerate of ductules with inter-twining myothelial proliferations constitutes a rounded structure of a highly characteristic appearance.

To the right, the same island at higher magnification.

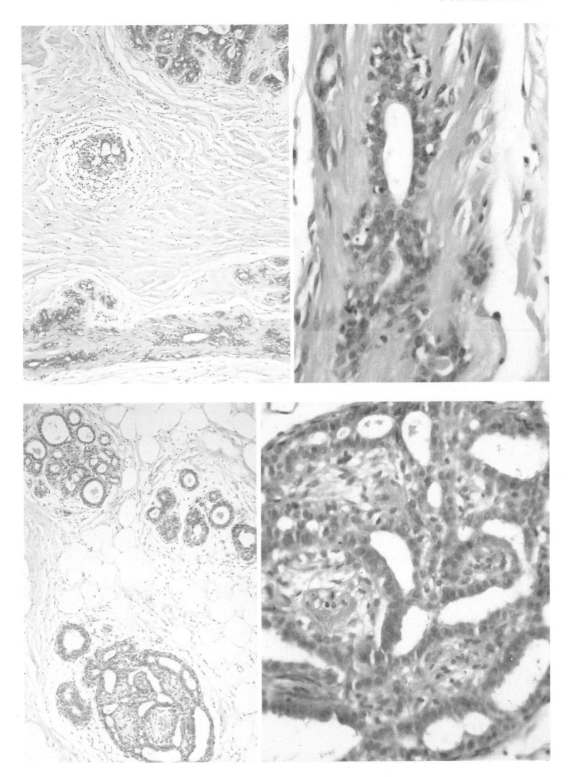

*Fig. 11-5*

*Clear cell lobules.* This is a rather rare finding. Occasionally lobules are encountered where the cells have a light "empty" cytoplasm and conspicuous cell borders. They resemble cells of a renal carcinoma. The cells have been called lamprocytes (from lampros, Gr. Light).

The clarity of the cytoplasm cannot be explained by the presence of fat or mucin. Nothing is known about their nature. As far as we know these cells have no pathologic importance but it may be worthwhile to be acquainted with their appearance.

To the left, a lobule exclusively made up of clear cells, but the connecting duct has normal appearing epithelium.

To the right, another lobule showing the light, slightly foamy cytoplasm of these lamprocytes.

*Fig. 11-6*

*"Satellite ducts".* This is the normal appearance of ducts surrounded by characteristic mantles of specialized stroma. The milk ducts (sinus) in the mammilla have star-shaped or crenelated lumina. In the breast tissue many ducts assume exaggerated forms of this appearance and satellite ducts will appear. On cross-section such satellite ducts may look like expansions from the central lumen (see the duct in the upper left). But very often the connection with the central lumen may be obliterated and the satellite ducts are seen running as parallel channels along the main ducts (see lower part left). By making multiple sequential sections Hamperl showed that the satellite ducts often anastomose with the main ducts. As Hamperl has remarked, the channel system in the female breast is constructed like some wine and liquor bottles.

To the right, a duct with many satellite ducts entering a lobule.

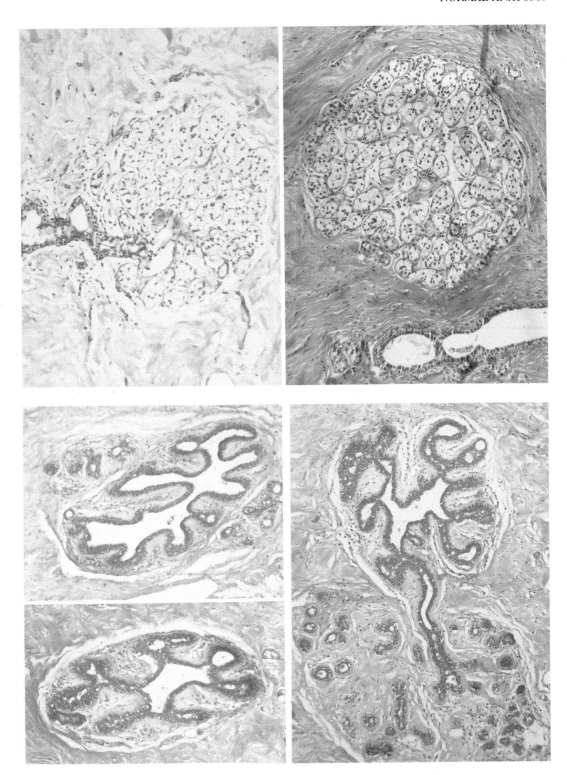

*Fig. 11-7*

*"Satellite ducts"*. The picture shows some ducts to give a more detailed illustration of satellite ducts. A 43-year-old woman.

To the left, satellite ducts with epithelium lining, continuous with the central channel.

To the right, a cross-section showing completely separated satellite ducts. In both pictures the epithelium and the myothelium appear as clearly separate layers.

In obliterative mastitis, causing obliteration of the main lumina of the ducts, which may be completely filled with granulation tissue, reactive epithelial proliferation from the satellite ducts is often a conspicuous feature (see Ch. 14).

*Fig. 11-8*

*Secretory lobule*. Such a change can be a remnant of lactation but one must be very cautious not to diagnose preceding lactation without anamnestic data. Such secretory changes, probably in some way hormonally influenced, may be seen even in women who have never been pregnant. These conditions have been excellently analyzed by Kiaer & Andersen.

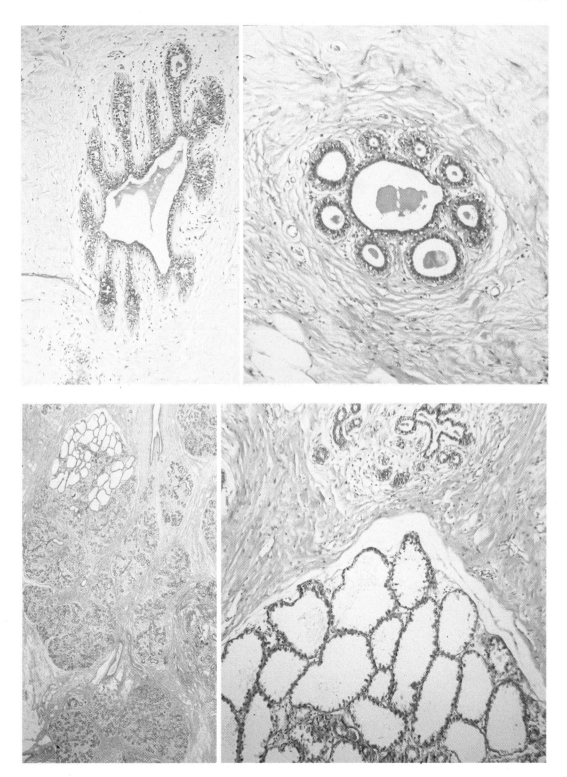

*Fig. 11-9*

*Cyclic changes*, correlated to the menstrual cycle, do exist in the breast tissue. They have been studied rather extensively, recently especially by Vogel et al. These authors claim that it is possible to characterize 5 different phases during the menstrual cycle. However, the human breast shows great variations and the cyclical changes are not always manifest in all parts of the breast tissue. Vogel et al. also admit that it is necessary to study many slides with good fixation to be able to detect the subtle changes due to hormonal changes during the menstrual cycle. We refer to the work of Vogel et al. and show only a few examples.

The figure shows breast tissue from a 16-year-old girl on the 7th day of her menstrual cycle. There ought to be no real stratification of the epithelium. Mitoses are a characteristic sign in this phase (arrow). Loose cellular stroma is also characteristic as well as tight acinar lumina without secretion.

But in this case the myothelial cells are conspicuous and there is secretion in the lumina, features which are said to be characteristic of the secretory phase of the cycle. The case illustrates that the picture does not always fit into the scheme.

*Fig. 11-10*

*Breast during menstrual cycle.* Menstrual phase (days 28 – 2). From a 26-year-old woman on her second cycle day. The tubules are open. Vacuolated myothelial cells are still present. The stroma is cellular and often contains mononuclear inflammatory cells. The picture shows also the variation that can be found. The lobule to the right is much more sclerotic.

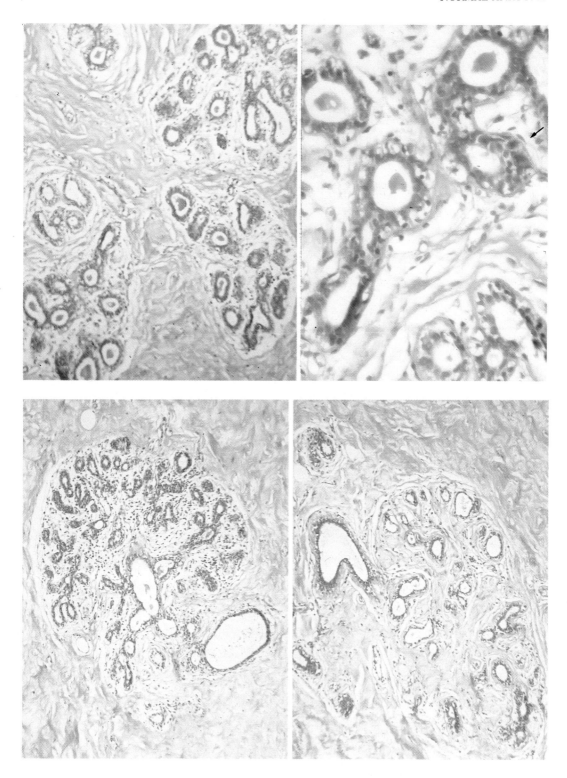

*Fig. 11-11*

*Aldactone induced proliferation.* An 85-year-old woman, who would normally have had very atrophic parenchyma. In this case, however, we see ducts and developing lobules with rather high epithelium. This woman has been treated with aldactone. From male cases (see Fig. 18 – 3) we know that aldactone very often produces gynecomastia. In women such proliferation will easily be overlooked or misinterpreted. We do not know whether aldactone has any carcinogenic properties.

*Fig. 11-12*

*Breast tissue during pregnancy.* During pregnancy profound changes occur in the mammary tissue. There are lively epithelial proliferations, leading to a breakdown of connective tissue, gradually substituted by densely packed, large lobules with outgrowth of small ramifications, i.e. the true acini, which are seen only in pregnancy and lactation.

The pictures are from a 21-year-old woman in the middle of her pregnancy. Left: In the lower part, densely packed large lobules, and in the upper part, still large fibrotic areas with ducts and atrophic lobules.

Right: Packed lobules with narrow septa between them. The cells are vacuolated.

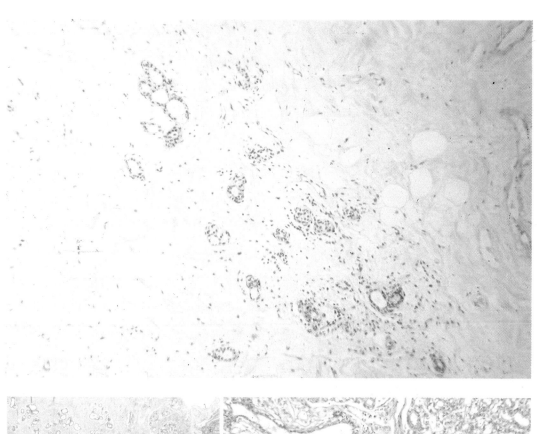

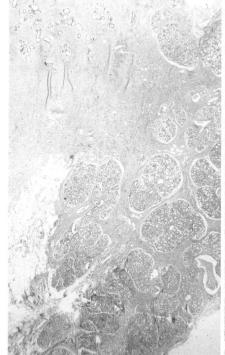
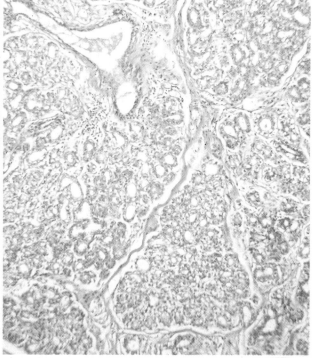

*Fig. 11-13*

*Breast tissue during lactation.* From a 37-year-old woman, who died 3 hours after her first partus from a bleeding complication. Her breasts were large and tense and yellow milk oozed from the cut surfaces.

To the left, densely packed large lobules with narrow connective tissue septa. But to the right we see persisting fibrous parts with few lobules and dilated ducts.

*Fig. 11-14*

*Breast tissue during lactation.* The same case as the foregoing.

To the left, densely packed lobules with very thin septa and vacuolated cells lining the open acini.

To the right a high-power field showing the vacuolated cells in the acini. There is no distinct layering of the cells.

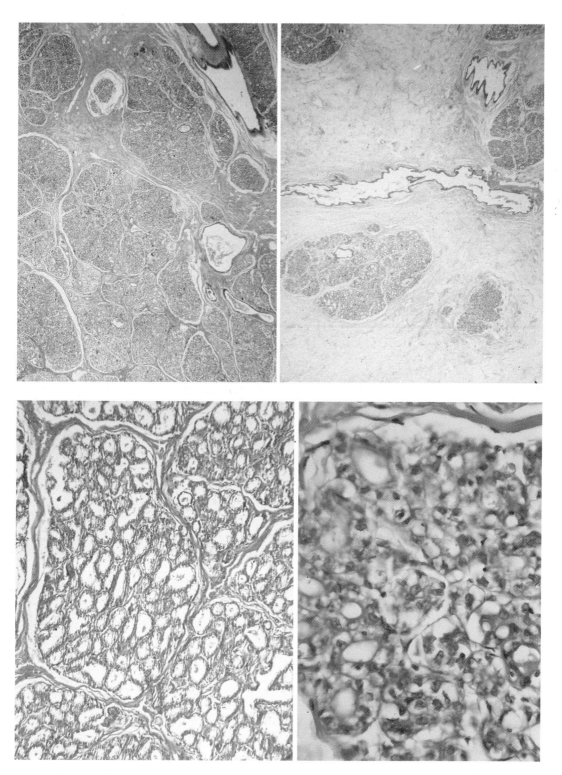

*Fig. 11-15*

*Breast tissue during lactation.* From a young woman who was still lactating 13 months after partus.

Left: On the right, there are densely packed lobules in full secretion and on the left, a well demarcated fibroadenoma (see Ch. 13) with no signs of secretion. This is not the rule as during lactation fibroadenomas may show areas of secretion.

Center: Secretory lobules with dilated acini.

Right: At high magnification, hobnail-shaped cells lining the acini. The myothelial cells are inconspicuous.

*Fig. 11-16*

*Macromastia in pregnancy.* On rare occasions during pregnancy, and sometimes even after pregnancy, a grotesque macromastia may develop. Sometimes the changes regress after interruption of pregnancy. The breast may grow to a weight of several kilograms (Leis & Östberg).

The picture is from the previously published case. Interestingly, the macromastia is not caused by secretory changes. The picture shows densely packed lobules which can be rather sclerotic. In many cases large reduction plasties must be resorted to.

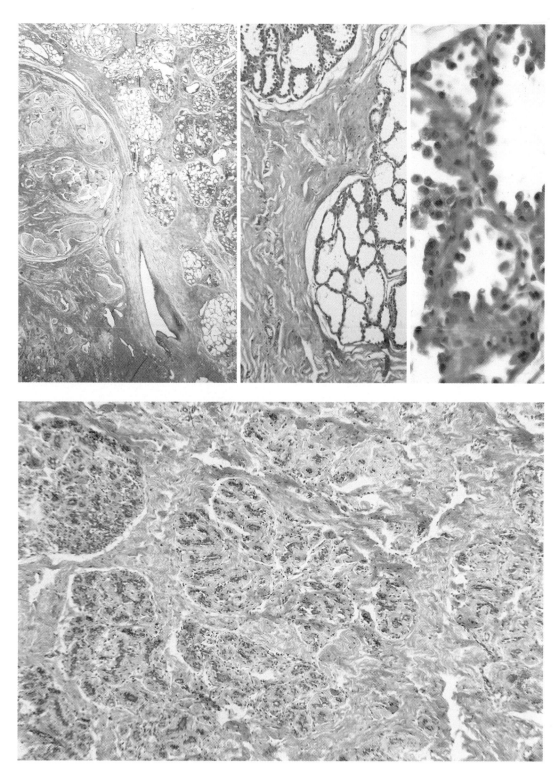

*Fig. 11-17*

*Involution of breast tissue.* A series of pictures of breast tissue derived from the same woman, showing involution. To the left, the breast at the age of 38. In the center, 6 years later. During this time there is no detectable change. The breast tissue contains a large number of normal lobules.

To the right, at the age of 49, we see the pronounced change that has taken place during the last 5 years. The number of lobules is markedly reduced and the relative amount of fat tissue has increased.

This process of involution may show great variation in different individuals. The involution is mostly far more pronounced in individuals who have borne children early. The process of involution is slower in the nulliparous and in women having their first children late. This is especially evident in mammographic studies (Wolfe et al.).

*Fig. 11-18*

*"Normal fat involution".* During aging there are involutionary processes leading to an increase in fatty tissue and an atrophy of the breast parenchyma. This process can vary in extent and be very heterogenous in different women. This has been known for a long time by pathologists but has not been fully appreciated until mammography came into common use. It is quite certain that the involutionary processes are mostly more rapid in women having had children at an early age and/or many children. Nulliparous women or women having had their first child when rather old will retain much more breast parenchyma.

To the left, breast tissue consisting mostly of fatty tissue with very thin strands of connective tissue with a few lobules and ducts. To the right, a detail with a duct with epithelium surrounded by a very conspicuous myothelium. We often meet these pictures in women more than 60 years old, and very occasionally in much younger women also.

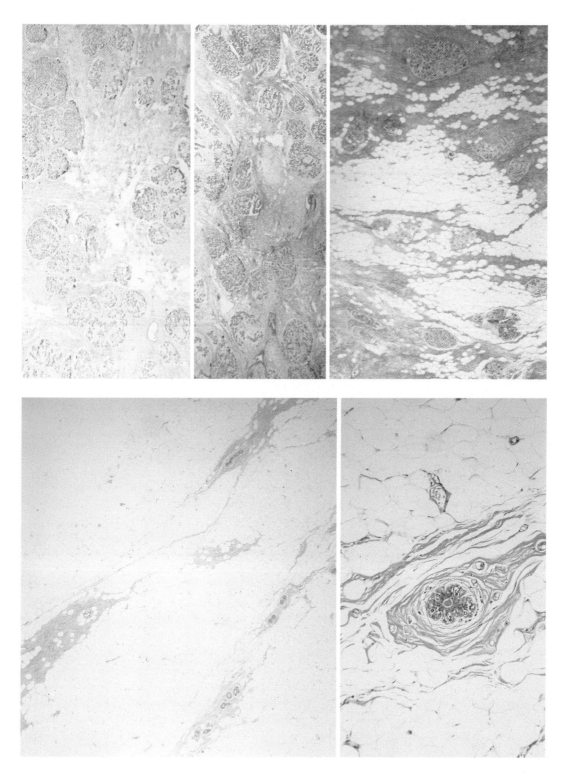

*Fig. 11-19*

*Naked lobules in fatty tissue*. Lobules are mostly situated in a more or less prominent connective tissue stroma. Now and then, however, one encounters lobules which are lying naked in the fatty tissue.

Left: At the top, breast tissue with connective tissue strands containing many lobules and, at the bottom, fatty tissue with scattered lobules devoid of intervening stroma. Right: Detail of a lobule lying "naked" in the adipose tissue. This picture may be encountered at all ages and seems to be a normal phenomenon.

In "adenolipomas" (see Ch. 13-14) "naked" lobules lying in adipose tissue is a conspicuous finding.

*Fig. 11-20*

*Lobular involution*. From a 49-year-old woman. To the left, a large lobule with marked fibrosis and *rarefaction* of end tubules.

To the right, a fibrous mass with only one end tubule, suggesting a remnant of a lobule in the fibrotic island. Lobules, however, can also vanish, leaving no vestiges.

As mentioned previously, this process can be seen at all ages but clearly, it is first of all an aging process. Most women have fatty involution and the parenchyma vanishes progressively. In this process the lobules disappear first; the ducts persist much longer. The ducts are often surrounded by hyaline connective tissue mantles.

Sometimes the lobular involution may be cystic in type (not shown here), whereby the end tubules dilate and form microcysts. This process may be interpreted as an early stage in the development of cystic breast disease which is, however, considered a distinct process. Indeed, it may be impossible to distinguish between these two conditions, especially as both may occur together in the same breast.

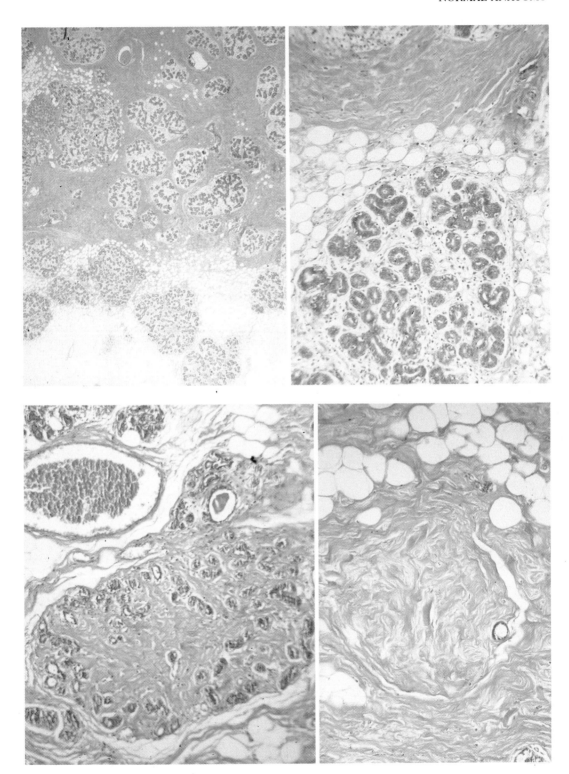

*Fig. 11-21*

*Normal "fibrosis".* The designation "fibrosis mammae" is often used by pathologists, probably even more so, earlier. Many women visit their doctor because of some kind of lump, often ill-defined. Very often these "lumps" are removed because the patient is anxious or the doctor is uncertain about their nature. In such cases the pathologist often finds no abnormalities either macroscopically or microscopically. The pathologist is mostly a "polite" person and feels inclined to give some explanation for or description of the subjective or clinical finding. He tends to avoid use of the diagnosis "normal mammary tissue". Instead "fibrosis mammae", an empty and insignificant designation, will most often be used and the pathologist, the clinician and the patient will all be satisfied.

In earlier days, before mammography and fine needle aspiration, "lumps" were excised consisting of what could honestly be called normal variants of breast tissue.

To the left, mammary tissue from a 38-year-old woman with rather few ducts and lobules, often called "interlobular" fibrosis. To the right, a detail of a lobule with "intralobular" fibrosis, which in reality represents involution, a feature that can be seen at all ages.

*Fig. 11-22*

*Involution in anorexia nervosa.* We have seen this in two cases. The picture shows breast tissue from a 34-year-old woman. In the connective tissue ducts are often seen surrounded by a loose myxomatous tissue. But there are no lobules. The picture exactly duplicates that of gynecomastia (compare Ch. 18 – 1-2). It seems that the inanition has initiated an atrophy of the parenchyma starting with involution of lobules. This process appears to be essentially the same as the normal physiologic involution.

Right: A detail (arrow pointing to the left).

In this case local excisions has been performed seven times during the last 9 years and the picture has invariably been the same. The patient has used contraceptive pills for many years.

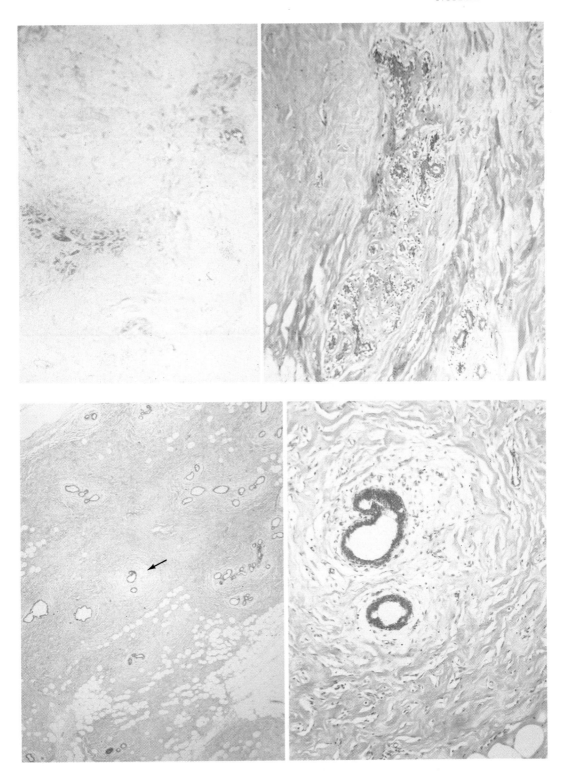

*Fig. 11-23*

*Fibrosis after radiation.* A 41-year-old woman, who was operated on in her left breast for an infiltrating comedo carcinoma. A quadrant excision was done and the rest of the breast irradiated (50 Grey). Fifteen months later a recurrence in the scar tissue was excised and 15 months later a bilateral subcutaneous mastectomy was performed. The breasts were small (right 100 g, left 80 g). The left breast was fibrotic.

The picture shows sections through the two breasts. To the right, the right breast showing parenchyma with ducts and lobules. Some of the lobules showed cribriform atypia.

To the left, the left breast with a pronounced fibrosis, leaving only a few atrophic remnants of ducts and lobules. This is the picture 3 years after the radiation.

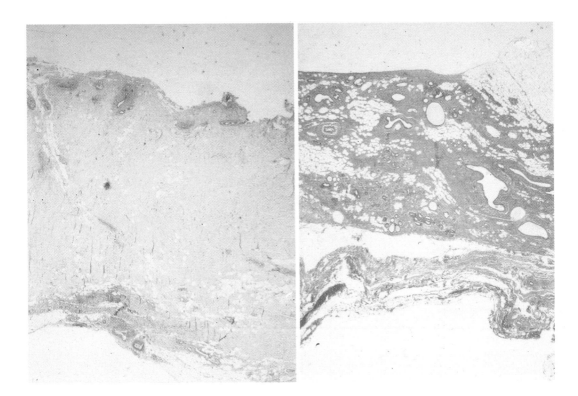

*Chapter 12*

# Inflammatory Changes

*Fig. 12-1*

*Unspecific mastitis.* This is a case of abscess-forming mastitis.

To the left, a picture of the breast tissue. The normal structures (ducts and lobules) have been destroyed and are replaced by a granulation tissue, richly vascularized and infiltrated by numerous inflammatory cells.

Though not found in this particular case, purulent mastitis is often a complication of lactation and usually develops during the first few weeks after parturition. The most common pathogen is Staphylococcus aureus, which gives rise to abscess formation. The process is usually confined to one lobe of the breast but may sometimes be multifocal. Nowadays, the natural course of the infection is usually interrupted by antibiotic therapy. Beta-hemolytic streptococci may occasionally cause a mastitis which tends to be more widespread or phlegmonous in type and associated with a marked regional lymphadenitis and general toxemia. Non-purulent infective mastitis may occur as a result of various viral infections.

To the right, widespread destruction of the normal elements, and development of granulomas with histiocytes and giant cells. This should not arouse suspicion of specific inflammation. Breast tissue contains a large amount of fat and during its breakdown histiocytes and giant cells accumulate. Oil cysts may develop, often surrounded by giant cells. Thus we may find a gradual transition towards inflammatory processes of a pronounced granulomatous character.

*Fig. 12-2*

*"Mild unspecific mastitis".* The picture shows a very common phenomenon that is often overlooked, probably quite rightly. The patient, a 72-year-old woman, had felt a lump in her breast but had no other complaints. The surgical specimen showed no macroscopic changes.

Histologically the breast parenchyma is seen to be fibrous and atrophic.

Left: At the bottom, a dilated duct connected with some small lobules with scattered lymphocytes.

Right: At the lower right, a lobule with extensive destruction and disappearance of end tubules and a persisting lymphocytic infiltrate (arrow).

Changes of the type seen in this picture mostly have no clinical correlation. They are coincidental findings in tissue which happens to be studied. In our opinion these small lymphocytic infiltrates are reactive changes in connection with physiological involution of breast tissue and are to be looked upon as normal findings.

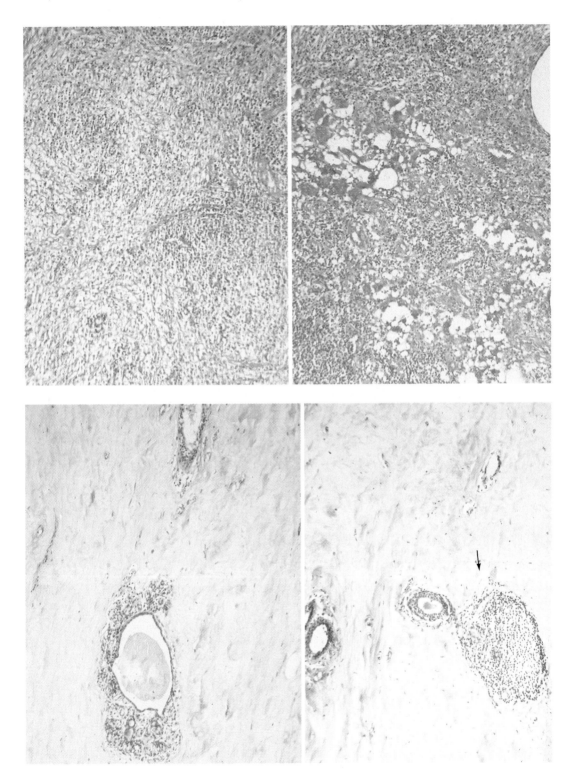

*Fig. 12-3*

*Granulomatous mastitis.* This condition is a recently defined entity of unknown etiology and pathogenesis which by definition (Kessler & Wolloch, 1972) is unrelated to fat necrosis, tuberculosis, syphilis or other "specific" granulomatous diseases, sarcoidosis or obliterative mastitis. It seems mainly to affect young women. It usually presents as a lump in the breast which, by palpation, may easily be mistaken for a carcinoma. Nowadays, using fine needle aspiration, its inflammatory nature is usually disclosed preoperatively. In contrast to tuberculosis the lesions are typically confined to the lobules. The granulomas show no caseous necroses and may often contain neutrophils.

Left: Rounded granulomas, which have replaced lobules. The granulomas consist of epitheloid cells and a few giant cells. At the periphery there is sometimes a rim of lymphocytes. At the top, a granuloma with giant cells and a central oil cyst.

Right: Three granulomas, replacing lobules. The one at the bottom also shows a broad perifocal zone of round cells. Centrally, there is an admixture of leukocytes.

*Fig. 12-4*

*"Sarcoidosis in connection with carcinoma".* The patient had a hard tumor in her breast.

The picture shows part of an axillary node. To the left an area which is dominated by metastasis of carcinoma, here growing as undifferentiated columns. But scattered among the clusters of carcinoma cells there are epitheloid granulomas (arrows). A field with several granulomas all containing giant cells is seen in the picture to the right.

Contrary to this case, sarcoid reaction in lymph nodes regional to a carcinoma is most often found in nodes which do not contain metastases. For discussion on the pathogenesis of this reaction see *e.g.* Gorton & Linell. It should be realized that sarcoid granulomas in axillary lymph nodes in a case of breast carcinoma may represent a generalized sarcoidosis, a possibility which should be investigated.

Granulomatous disease of the breast was more common formerly, when it was frequently a manifestation of tuberculosis. Such lesions, as well as other infective granulomas, show no special features in the breast and the reader is referred to common books of infectious diseases.

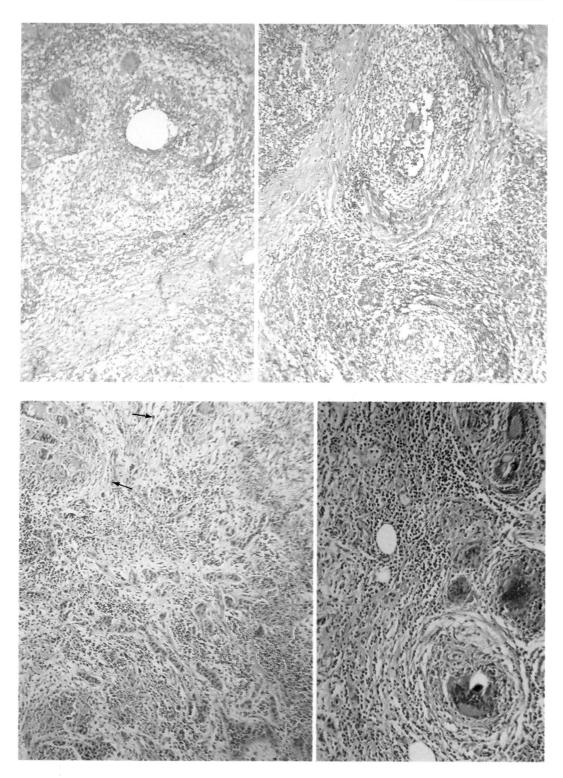

*Fig. 12-5*

*Retention mastitis with ductectasia*. The picture shows a case of cystic disease with dilated ducts containing foam cells and surrounded by round cells. Some degree of acute inflammation with admixture of leucocytes may also be seen.

Retention of secretions and desquamative products within the ducts is a common phenomenon, especially in elderly women. Moderate amounts of such material can easily be eliminated by resorption and passage to the surface via the ductal system. But when excessive amounts are formed or when any hindrance of the outflow through the nipple occurs, ductectasia may supervene with a more or less pronounced chronic inflammation. This form of chronic mastitis may clinically present as nodular or diffuse, rather hard lumps, sometimes misinterpreted as carcinoma. The condition may develop in glandular tissue which has previously been altered by various manifestations of cystic disease, described in more detail in Ch. 14.

Left: An area of cystic disease. An inflamed duct is seen (arrow).

Right: A detail with the inflamed duct filled with foam cells and leukocytes. In the surrounding tissue are many leukocytes and at the bottom right (arrow) an almost completely destroyed lobule.

*Fig. 12-6*

*Retention mastitis with ductectasia and foam cell granulomas*. The dilated ducts in retention mastitis accumulate a fluid which may be either thin and rather clear or thick and cream-like. In the latter case it consists of large numbers of foam cells, necrotic cells and cholesterol crystals.

To the left, ducts, whose epithelium is often more or less destroyed. The ducts contain deposits of cholesterol mixed with foam cells and brown-colored macrophages containing iron pigments and lipofuscin. A further stage in this process is the formation of foreign body granulomas.

Sometimes the ducts and their surroundings may be replaced by granulation tissue. To the right, a duct filled with foam cells. The borders of the duct can be seen (arrows) even if the epithelium has been destroyed. Periductally the same dense aggregations of foam cells are seen blended with less conspicuous round cell infiltrates.

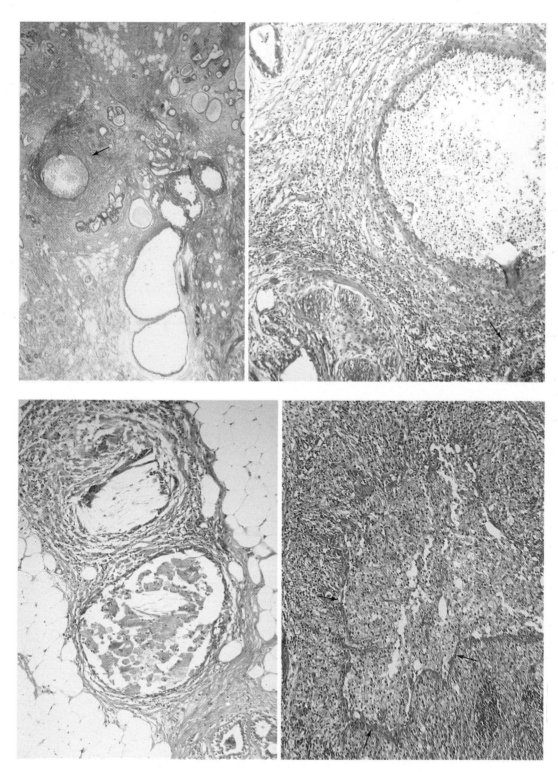

*Fig. 12-7*

*Retention mastitis with obliteration of ducts ("obliterative mastitis").* The picture shows a duct with regular epithelium, but part of the lumen is occupied by granulation tissue with foreign body giant cells, containing cholesterol crystals and histiocytes. Dystrophic calcification may occur in these deposits, as shown in Fig. 12 – 9. The peripheral part of the granulation "plug" shows beginning fibrosis. Outside and within this zone some epithelium-lined channels, seemingly in an active stage of proliferation, are seen. They are remnants of the "satellite" ducts (see Ch. 11 – 6-7).

Obliterative lesions of the ducts are treated in more detail in Ch. 14.

Obliterative lesions are common findings but not always appreciated. Mostly they are of little clinical significance.

*Fig. 12-8*

*"Plasma cell mastitis".* This name has been applied to a variant of the retention syndrome characterized by an admixture of plasma cells to the periductal round cell infiltrate. The milk ducts are dilated with retention of debris and there may be varying degrees of periductal fibrosis.

To the left, a general view with fibrous streaks containing dilated ducts with eosinophil retention products. The ducts have a wavy contour speaking for a shrinking process due to the periductal fibrosis. The ducts are surrounded by more or less continuous mantles of round cells. Clinically plasma cell mastitis is often described as a lumpy process in the central part of the breast with retractions of the skin and especially of the mammilla.

To the right, a detail showing the preserved epithelium and the inflammatory infiltrate with lymphocytes and rather few plasma cells.

After the introduction of mammography plasma cell mastitis has come to mean a special entity, somewhat different from classical plasma cell mastitis as defined by pathologists (see Fig. 12-9).

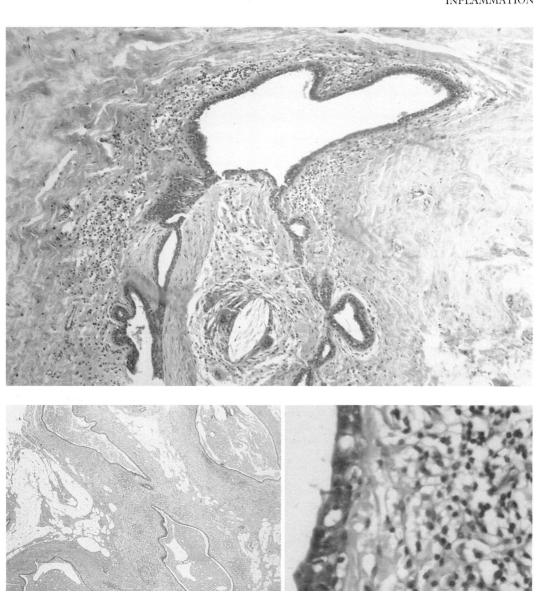

*Fig. 12-9*

*"Plasma cell mastitis" with pronounced calcifications.* By mammography "plasma cell mastitis" is described as having a pathognomonic X-ray picture, consisting of a bundle of dilated ducts which radiate from the mammilla and contain more or less continuous calcifications.

The picture to the left shows two dilated ducts with more or less preserved epithelium. The ducts contain debris with many calcifications of various sizes.

To the right, at a higher magnification, such a duct with calcified particles. In this case the epithelium is destroyed and the wall is thickened and partly hyalinized. No plasma cells are seen in this case, indicating that the term "plasma cell mastitis" is a misnomer for this condition. In fact, plasma cells are never a prominent feature and the name ought to be abandoned and replaced by the more neutral name "retention syndrome" to adequately cover all variants of the condition.

*Fig. 12-10*

*Ivalon prosthesis.* Different materials have been used to compensate for breast tissue either after operative removal or for augmentation of breasts too small for aestetic satisfaction or for sexual excitement (topless artists in shows). Ivalon was the prosthetic material most often used in early days (during the sixties). This material is rather hard and unnatural but can give a very good architectural exterior. Ivalon is a plastic material with numerous spaces that are initially filled with fluid which is later on organized by ingrowing connective tissue. This leaves very hard prostheses, which to the eye and the palpating fingers give the impression of a marble statue. Such hard prostheses are very disagreeable for the owner and this material has been abandoned, although a few such prostheses may still be in use.

The picture on the left shows a part of an ivalon prosthesis. The ivalon stains blue in hematoxy-lin-eosin and is built up by anastomosing, often triangle-shaped strands, embedded in ingrowing granulation tissue. To the left, a part of the hyaline connective tissue capsule is seen.

The picture to the right shows, at higher magnification, the blue ivalon strands, partly surrounded by fibrous tissue with numerous foreign body giant cells.

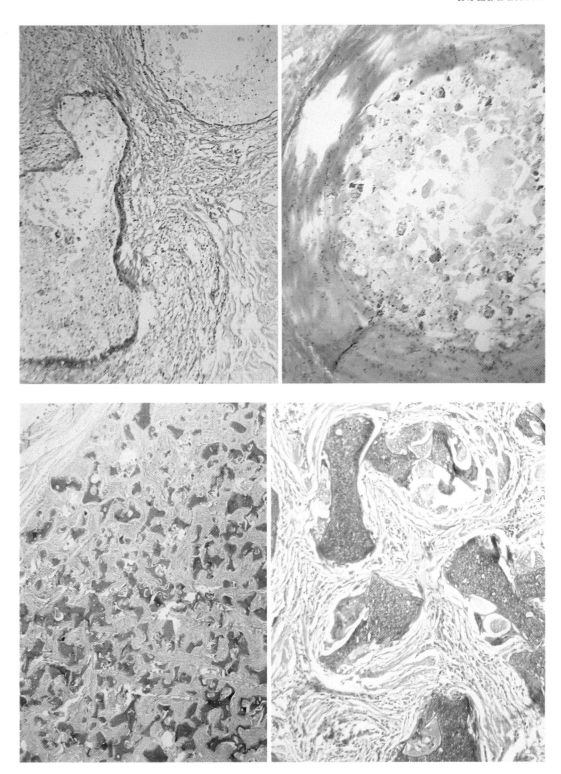

*Fig. 12-11*

*Silicone granuloma.* Silicone has also been used to augment breast tissue. In the beginning it was injected, with very bad results because it elicited a chronic foreign body inflammation.

Prostheses of silicone coated with a thin capsule has been used with good results, having a natural consistency, especially when they are inserted under the pectoral muscle. When placed subcutaneously, the prostheses sometimes become surrounded by hard connective tissue capsules, which felt hard and converted the prostheses to round bodies reminiscent of oranges. But silicone prostheses may rupture on violent handling, eliciting a foreign body inflammation in the surrounding tissue. Leakage through the capsule may also occur. The silicone may spread to the axillary lymph nodes. Histologically the reaction resembles the changes after lymphangiography with oily contrast.

The picture to the left shows granulation tissue after rupture into subcutaneous fatty tissue. In the granulation tissue there are numerous, apparently empty, rounded spaces.

The picture to the right shows these spaces filled with unstained silicone which can be visualized by using small aperture. Around the silicone particles are round cells, histiocytes and giant cells. In the center of the picture on the right there is a beautiful asteroid body in the hyaline cytoplasm of a multinucleated giant cell.

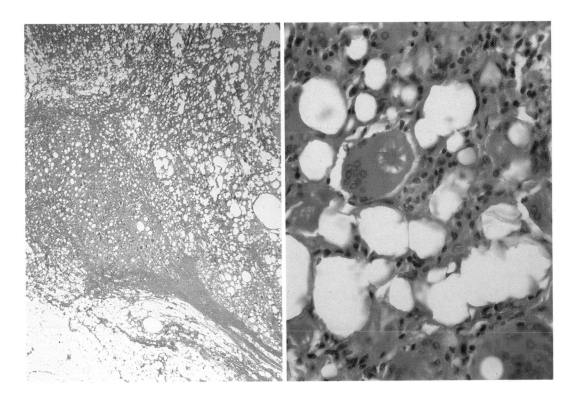

*Chapter 13*

# Benign Tumors and Tumor-like Lesions

*Fig. 13-1*

*Fibroadenoma.* This term designates an extremely common lesion in the female breast. In its typical form it is a well demarcated tumor measuring from 1 to 5-6 cm. It is common in teenagers, but the peak in clinical diagnostics is in the third or fourth decades. Fibroadenoma is usually a solitary tumor. On rare occasions it may be multiple and/or bilateral.

The pictures show a series of typical fibroadenomas. They are mostly well demarcated but often adherent to the surrounding tissue and therefore cannot always easily be shelled out. They are moderately firm and the cut surface is often bulging, lobulated and gelatinous and glistening. The macroscopic picture is mostly very typical but there are cases which are not readily recognized macroscopically. In the following, different types and variations in histology will be shown.

Microscopic fibroadenomas are extremely common. They may be found in practically every breast and are often multiple.

*Fig. 13-2*

*Fibroadenoma* (intracanalicular type). The picture shows part of the tumor. Upper part, sharply demarcated border. The typical histology shows ductal structures often extended as antlers. The epithelium is regular with two conspicuous layers. Especially in young persons the stroma is loose and myxomatous (see following pictures). The stroma often bulges into the glandular structures as papillomatous excrescences with regular epithelium. It is essential to notice that the fibroadenomatous structure can be described as a distortion of a normal lobule. In practically every breast one may find microscopic fibroadenomas which have arisen from single lobules or parts of lobules. Fibroadenomas are principally benign, although there are rare exceptions (Figs. 13-10 and 13-11).

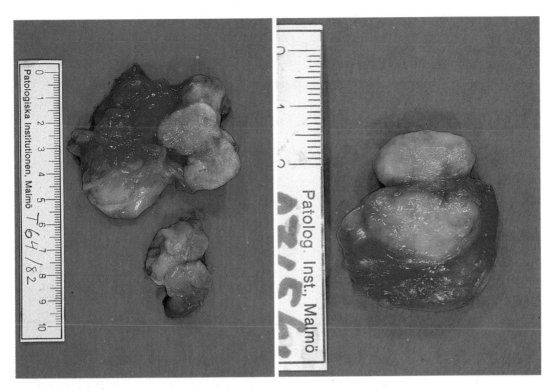

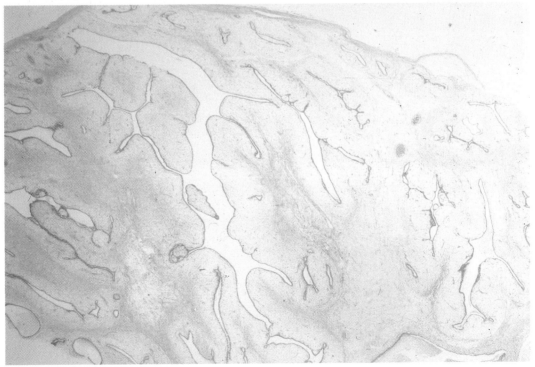

*Fig. 13-3*

*Fibroadenoma with pronounced myxomatous stroma.* This type of fibroadenoma is mostly seen in rather young patients. The stroma contains an increased amount of mucosubstances and fluid which makes the cut surfaces transparent and gives the tumor a myxomatoid character. This also results in an increased intratumoral pressure which is why the tumor tends to bulge on the cut surface and may feel rather hard on palpation.

To the left, the distorted ducts, often compressed with atrophic epithelium due to the swelling myxomatous stroma, having a few spindle-shaped cells in a mucous substance.

To the right, an Alcian-blue-PAS staining. The stroma stains blue due to acid mucosubstances. The ducts contain red-stained alkaline mucous material.

*Fig. 13-4*

*Juvenile fibroadenoma with cellular stroma.* This tumor is from a young woman. To the left, an overview with the antler-like ducts in an eosinophil, very cellular stroma. The demarcation from the surrounding tissue is seen in the upper part. Fibroadenomas have no true capsules.

To the right, at a higher magnification. The duct shows a high cylindric epithelium, rather basophil but regular. Only a few light myothelial cells can be seen. The stroma is cellular with many fibroblasts without atypia. No mitoses.

Juvenile fibroadenomas may grow rapidly and reach large dimensions ("giant" fibroadenoma). As in this case, they typically show a very cellular stroma with a marked myxoid character. A high degree of branching of the ducts and cleft formation may be a reminiscent of cystosarcoma phyllodes. But the tumor is wholly benign and has no relationship to cystosarcoma phyllodes (Ch. 16).

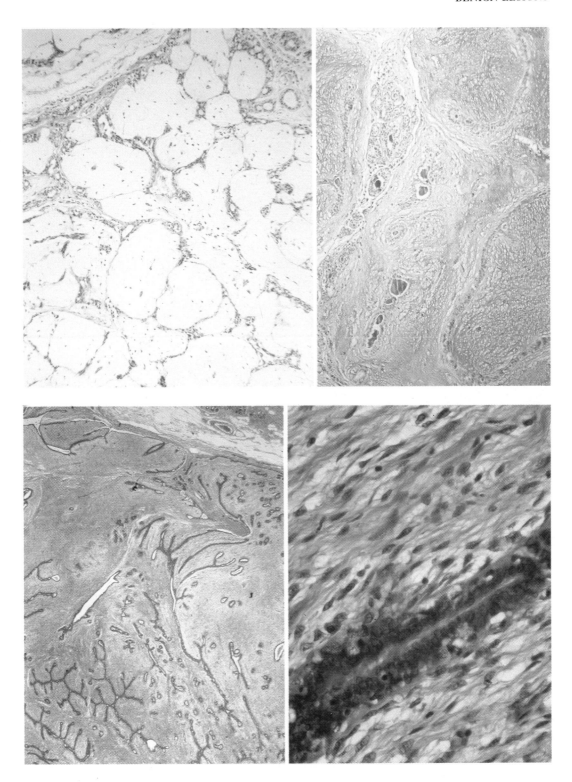

*Fig. 13-5*

*Fibroadenoma with unusual elastosis.* Rather small fibroadenoma with typical structure except a predominant amount of stroma with abundant deposits of elastic tissue. We have no explanation to offer for this feature. It is a very rare finding. Weigert's elastica stain.

*Fig. 13-6*

*Fibroadenoma with apocrine metaplasia.* The close relationship between the mammary lobule and the fibroadenoma is revealed by the occurrence of different lesions in fibroadenomas, which are identical to the various epithelial and myothelial changes seen in cystic breast disease (mastopathia cystica) and sclerosing adenosis. Left: In the upper part, the well demarcated border is seen and nearby irregular ducts with apocrine metaplasia. The lower part shows a more common variety of fibroadenoma pattern with myxomatous stroma.

Right: A high-power field of the same tumor. The upper part of the picture shows ducts with high papillary eosinophil epithelium of the same kind as in cystic lesions (compare Figs. 14 – 1-2). The lower part shows typical fibroadenoma with loose myxomatous stroma.

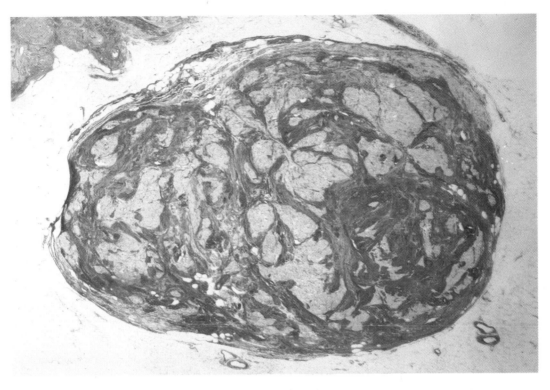

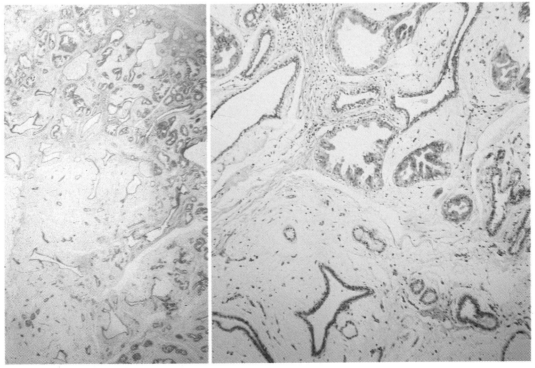

*Fig. 13-7*

*Fibroadenoma with epitheliosis.* This is also an example of a lesion seen in cystic disease but located in a fibroadenoma. Left: A clearly outlined border. In the lower part, ordinary fibroadenoma structures. Most of the tumor is occupied by ducts with high, often multi-layered, epithelium that often fills up the lumen. This is better seen in the picture to the right. The epithelial cells show small nucleoli and there is no real atypia. The lesion is wholly benign. We have seen the same type of change in different fibroadenomas removed from the same woman at intervals of several years.

A special type of epitheliosis has been thought to be composed of "endocrine" cells (Eusebi et al.). Right (arrow): Some cells with light cytoplasm. Such cells may contain argyrophil granules but this is no certain proof of an "endocrine" nature because argyrophilia may also be due to the presence of particles of lactalbumin.

*Fig. 13-8*

*Fibroadenoma with lobular carcinoma in situ.* Fibroadenomas are essentially benign tumors but on rare occasions they may show carcinomatous changes. The most common is the occurrence of lobular carcinoma in situ within ducts of the fibroadenoma. Usually the ducts of the fibroadenoma are involved by lobular carcinoma in situ, which is also present in the neighboring parenchyma. Whether this phenomenon represents an invasion into the fibroadenoma ducts by carcinoma cells from neighboring tubulo-lobular units or is a true in situ change within the fibroadenoma is difficult to prove. Occasionally, however, the change is apparently primary, i.e. found exclusively within the ducts of the fibroadenoma.

Left: The well demarcated fibroadenoma with a rather ordinary pattern in the lower part. The upper part shows the tubules filled with compact formations of epithelium.

Right: A higher magnification showing tubules filled with compact formations of rather small uniform cells (compare with Ch. 15).

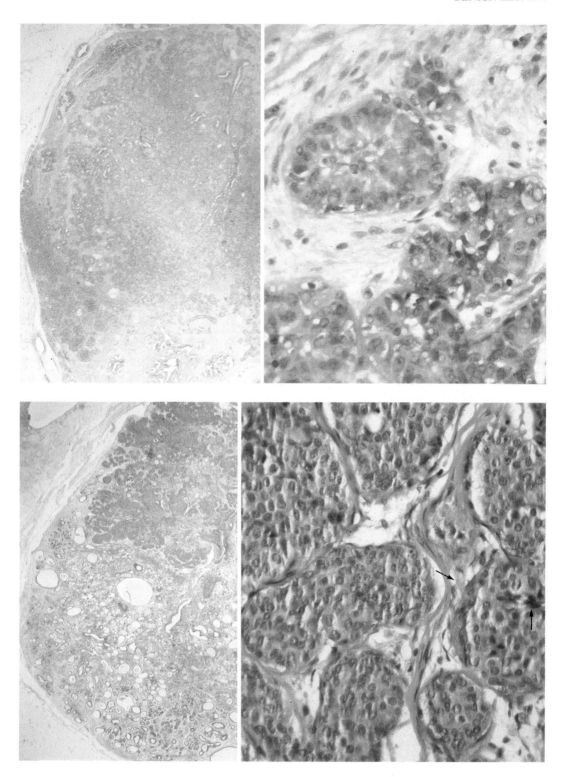

*Fig. 13-9*

*Fibroadenoma with intraductal carcinoma of comedo type.* This is a very rare event. Both primary and secondary invasion may occur; the latter variant seems to be the most common.

Left: A well demarcated fibroadenoma with mainly a rather ordinary fibroadenoma pattern. On the right there is more pronounced epithelial proliferation and some small lymphocytic infiltrates (arrow) can be seen.

Right: Higher magnification shows the multi-layered irregular and highly atypical epithelium. A mitosis (arrow) can be seen. In the stroma a sparse plasmocellular infiltration. In this case there was also intraductal carcinoma in the neighborhood of the fibroadenoma.

*Fig. 13-10*

*"Pure adenoma".* This lesion is considered in this connection, although it is uncertain if it really has anything common with fibroadenomas. Pure adenomas are mostly seen during pregnancy or lactation. They are well demarcated, several centimeters wide. On the cut surfaces they are grayish, grayish-yellow or, when occurring during lactation, cream-yellow, the yellow component being related to the degree of secretion and retention of secretory products.

The pictures are from a yellow tumor that was easily shelled out from the breast tissue of a 21-year-old woman in the fifth month of pregnancy.

To the left, the sharp border, delineated from the surrounding tissue by a thin layer of fatty tissue (compare with the hamartomas). The mass is composed of tightly packed tubules giving an impression of a very compact tumor.

To the right, a higher magnification of the tubules lined by vacuolated epithelium. The myothelial cells are few and difficult to discern. The tubules appear highly differentiated and closely resemble normal lobular end tubules. The stroma is sparse and, in contrast to that of fibroadenomas, the epithelial component is the sole neoplastic constituent of the tumor.

There is reason to believe that pure adenomas are related to hamartomas, described in Figs. 13-11-14 being hamartomas modified by pregnancy. Some may be fibroadenomas which, likewise, have been altered by changes during pregnancy.

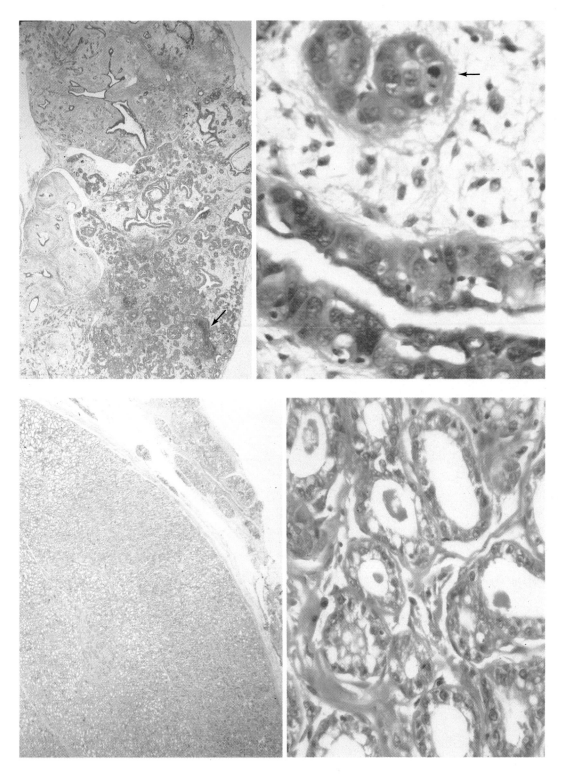

*Fig. 13-11*

*Hamartoma.* This is an entity that has not been appreciated until recent years (see references). Hamartomas are characterized as nonencapsulated tumor-like lesions. They are well demarcated by a thin layer of fatty tissue. They are composed of essentially normal mammary tissue and do not have the typical structure of fibroadenomas. They may vary in size from 1-2 cm up to about 20 cm and may weigh as much as 1500 g. They have a characteristic mammographic picture. They can surgically be shelled out very easily without bleeding, leaving behind an amount of breast tissue equal to that of the contralateral breast. When very large and rapidly growing they are easily recognized. But even rather large hamartomas can go unnoticed by the woman and by the doctor. They have mostly the same consistency as the surrounding mammary tissue and are thus not easily palpable.

The picture shows a hamartoma weighing 1000 g from a 13-year-old girl. She had her menarche 1 year earlier. Nine months later the girl noticed that one of her breasts was growing quickly. Initially she was rather proud of it but later she became afraid and tried to hide her situation. Three months later she came to the surgeon and the tumor-like lesion was easily shelled out.

To the left, the hamartoma is seen from the outside with its smooth, glistening surface. To the right, the cut surface with a grayish-yellow color and normal mammary tissue structure (compare the fibroadenomas in Fig. 13-1 with their white gelatinous bulging surfaces).

*Fig. 13-12*

*Hamartoma.* This is the microscopic picture of the lesion in Fig. 13-1. In the upper part its sharp delimitation is readily recognized. This is the most characteristic feature of the lesion. Another characteristic feature is its histologic structure, composed of normal-looking mammary tissue. In this case the lesion consists of juvenile breast tissue, mostly ducts and very little branching into lobules, and a loose stroma outlining the developing lobules. Kronsbein and Bässler have given an excellent description of the relation between the structure of the lesion and the patient's age.

To the right, a detail showing that the stroma can be rather well vascularized and hyaline between the lobules.

Hamartomas of this type seem to have first been described by Prym in 1928, but they have since been more fully characterized by Hogeman and Östberg (1968) and in several later papers (see references). Hamartomas of moderate size are easily overlooked by the patient, the clinician and especially by the pathologist. The macroscopic appearance is the only trait of the lesion which is really diagnostic. When the surgeon does not realize the nature of the lesion and excises only a piece of it, the pathologist is unable to diagnose the lesion correctly and the case may come to rest under the meaningless heading "fibrosis mammae" (cf. Ch. 2).

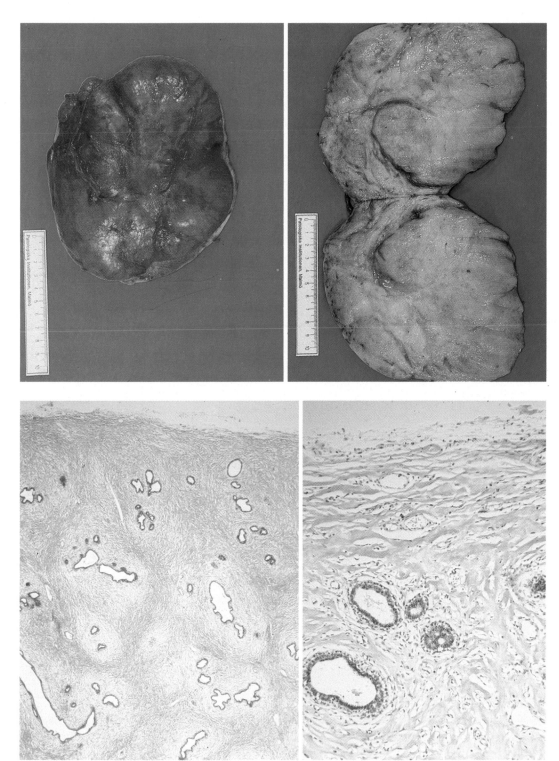

*Fig. 13-13*

*Hamartoma.* This is a very typical example illustrating how easily a hamartoma can be overlooked. This case was a 42-year-old woman who had borne three children and now underwent reduction mastoplasty whereby about 1000 g of mammary tissue was removed from each side. The surgeon did not notice anything peculiar but when the pathologist incised the large specimen he came across a hamartoma of about 7×6×3 cm, which popped up from the cut surface and could easily be shelled out. To the left, the hamartoma residing in its cave and surrounded by rather lipomatous mammary tissue.

To the right, the cut surface of the hamartoma. Notice the structural differences between this lesion and fibroadenomas in Fig. 13-1.

*Fig. 13-14*

*Hamartoma.* This is a further example illustrating the features described in the foregoing. The smooth outer contour is seen on the right in both pictures. Its histologic structure is built up of ordinary breast tissue with ducts and lobules. The stroma may be abundant and often sclerosed, as seen in the picture on the left.

Right: An area of adipose tissue. This is often seen and in some cases the fatty tissue may be the dominant ingredient of the lesion. This variant of hamartoma seems to correspond to the *adenolipomas,* described by Spalding. (cf. Ch. 11-19).

On rare occasions the breast tissue within hamartomas may show different types of changes (cystic disease, apocrine metaplasia, sclerosing adenosis) described in Ch. 14. For further discussion of these problems see Linell *et al.* (1979).

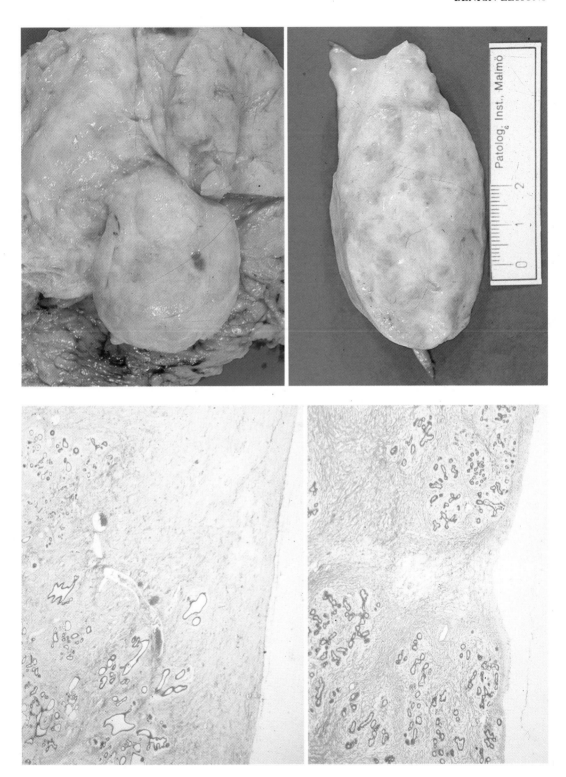

*Fig. 13-15*

*Intraductal papilloma*. Intraductal papilloma may be solitary or multiple. It is a common view that solitary papilloma is always benign whereas multiple papillomas ("papillomatosis") indicate a certain risk for the development into carcinoma. In reality we cannot make the distinction between solitary and multiple papillomas unless the whole breast is serially sectioned. This situation is practically never present when discussing the patient's risk. Therefore we must adhere to the common histologic and cytologic criteria for malignancy.

The papillomas often exhibit circulatory disturbances with infarctions and bleeding. Bloody secretion from the mammilla is usually a sign of a benign papilloma and rarely of a carcinoma.

To the left, a part of an intraductal papilloma with widespread hyalinization probably due to compromised circulation; papillomas often have very narrow stalks which can easily be twisted or compressed.

To the right, a well preserved part of the same papilloma. The epithelium is highly differentiated with regular nuclei. There is no suspicion of malignancy histologically.

*Fig. 13-16*

*Intraductal papilloma*. It is often stated, although without any reliable evidence, that an intraductal papilloma having a distinct stalk of connective tissue stroma is benign. Such a statement cannot be true in all cases. Evaluation of papillomas must also take into consideration other features such as cytologic atypia and cellular orientation.

The picture illustrates intraductal papillomas with an "adenomatous" pattern of gland-like structures in a fibrous stroma. As seen in the picture on the right there is little atypia; these papillomas are to be viewed as benign.

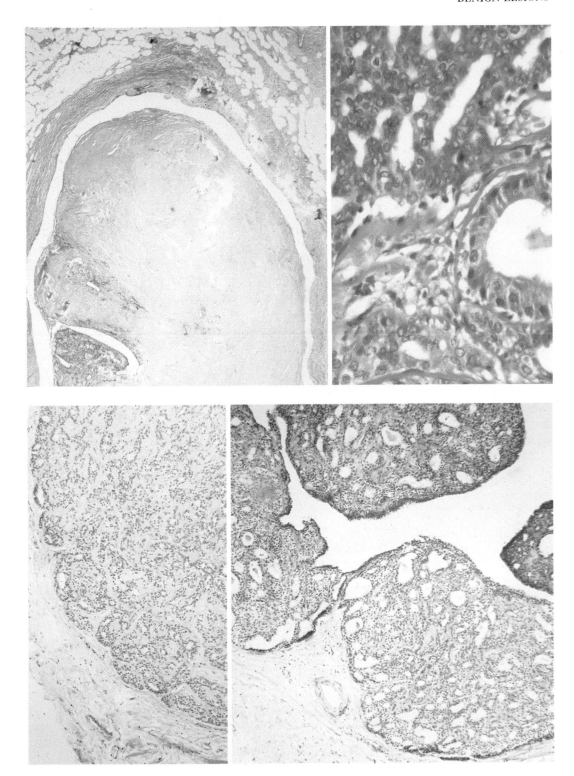

*Fig. 13-17*

*"Extreme juvenile papillomatosis"*. Very occasionally one encounters lumps in young women, often teenagers, showing vigorous papillomas, sometimes combined with other proliferative lesions. Some of these patients show up with carcinomas, often at a young age (Kiaer et al., 1979).

This picture shows breast tissue from a woman who was operated on because of relapsing lumps in her breasts, beginning at the age of 17. The lumps showed the same picture for 11 years at which time a bilateral subcutaneous mastectomy was performed.

Left: At the top, dilated ducts with vigorous papillomas. At the bottom, an area reminiscent of a large hyperplastic lobule. Right: Fibroadenomatous structures intermingled with large intraductal papillomas.

*Fig. 13-18*

*"Extreme juvenile papillomatosis"*. The picture represents another case, earlier published by Kiaer et al. (1979). This was a 46-year-old woman. This specimen was excised when she was 11 years old.

To the left, a picture of dilated ducts filled with papillomatous excrescences. The picture is extremely active and proliferative.

To the right, at a higher magnification. A certain degree of atypia is conspicuous. Mitoses are seen. Twenty-seven years later the woman developed invasive carcinoma. There seems to be good reason to take those pictures in young women seriously and to institute an active therapy or very close observation. This woman died from metastases at 46.

90

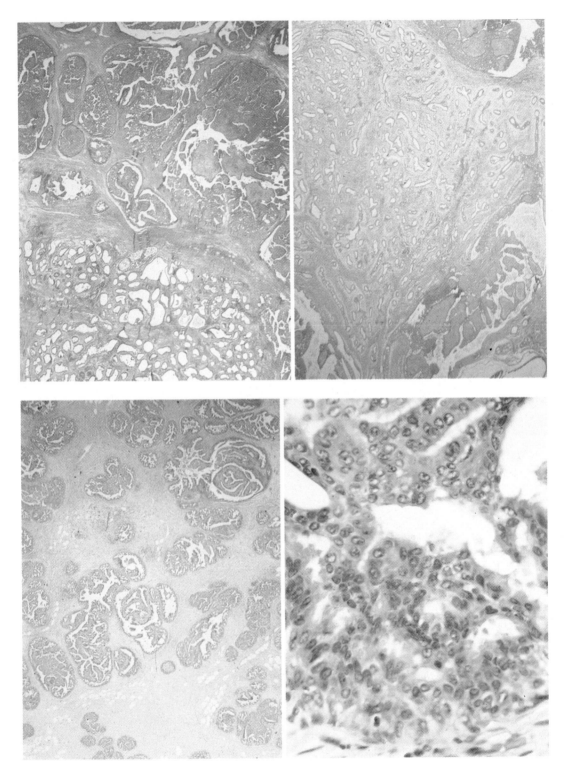

*Fig. 13-19*

*"Juvenile papillomatosis"* (Swiss cheese disease). This name has been used for some lesions which according to our opinion do not always merit the name "juvenile papillomatosis". Rosen et al. (1980) have described 33 cases and claim that these lesions have a characteristic macro- and microscopic pattern.

The picture shows such a lesion. A young woman with a rather circumscribed area of hard tissue with numerous cysts or holes reminiscent of Swiss cheese.

*Fig. 13-20*

*"Juvenile papillomatosis"* (Swiss cheese disease). This is the microscopic pattern, corresponding to the macroscopic picture (Fig. 13-19).

To the left, a lesion consisting of several groups of agglomerated cysts. Many of the cysts are "open" with a single layer of epithelium. Some, however, show more or less pronounced papillary foldings invard.

In the center, a group of cysts is seen with numerous papillary excrescences of large-celled apocrine epithelium.

To the right there is even more pronounced epitheliosis, papillary and solid. According to our opinion such pictures correspond to the pictures in the paper by Rosen et al. They have no specific or characteristic traits but fit in very well with what we see in cystic disease (see Ch. 14).

We feel that all features in the described lesions can be seen in fibrocystic disease. Rosen et al. claim that a characteristic feature is that the patients are young. This statement, however, is a circular proof because they chose their material from cases 30 years old or younger.

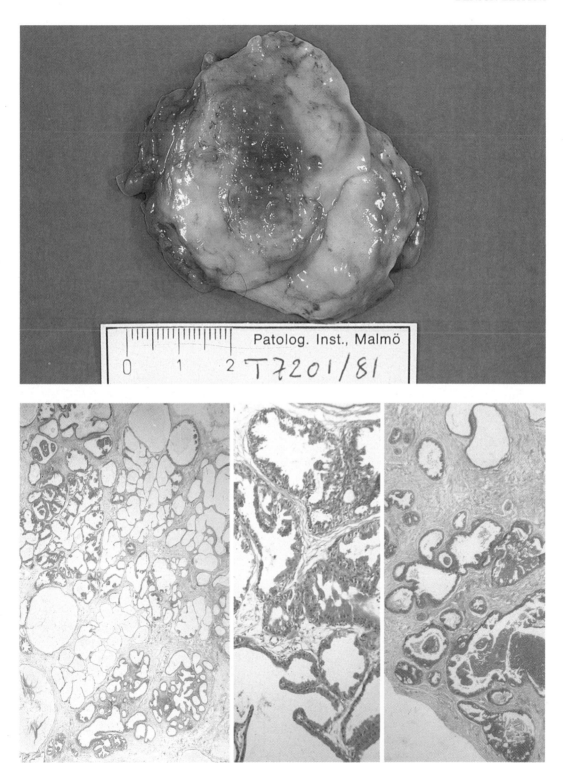

Patolog. Inst., Malmö

0 1 2 T7201/81

## Chapter 14

# Cystic Disease and Related Conditions

*Fig. 14-1*

*Cystic disease.* This name is used among many others (see Ch. 5) to denote a series of ill-defined clinical and histologic changes. Many of the pictures may be "normal" variations, but others are clearly proliferative changes, which may even constitute transitions towards neoplastic changes. In the following we will reproduce a sample of such changes.

This picture shows a very common finding which can be encountered at all ages. Most pathologists would call it cystic disease but when we see only small or few such changes in a specimen we tend to overlook them. We have no evidence that they represent any risk for malignancy.

To the left we see agglomerations of cysts with very thin walls lined by eosinophil papillary epithelium of apocrine type. The cells are large, granulated and of oncocytic type. Such cysts are often interpreted as dilated ducts but they are more probably altered lobular structures, as their lobular arrangement suggests.

Structures of this type are encountered in practically every breast extensively studied histologically. When the changes are pronounced they may give rise to nodules in the breast. We are inclined to view such instances as pathologic.

There are good reasons to believe that the different pictures seen in this condition are the result of proliferation and involution, which, in turn, have their basis in an abnormality of hormonal stimuli and stromal and epithelial response. The structural alteration of the breast tissue may be very unevenly distributed and may result in more or less pronounced deviations from what we call normal.

*Fig. 14-2*

*Epitheliosis in cystic disease.* The changes hitherto described in this chapter have an apparently benign character but we often encounter changes which may arouse suspicion of being premalignant. Mostly the changes are characterized by epithelial proliferation. These proliferations, often called epitheliosis, mostly show very little epithelial atypia but we do not know if they are an early step on the way to neoplastic development. There are studies indicating that such epitheliosis indicates a higher degree of risk for developing malignancy (3-4 fold risk according to McDivitt). Compare the picture with Rosen's juvenile papillomatosis (Fig. 13 – 19-20). In reality there are no differences between Swiss cheese disease and the proliferative changes in cystic disease.

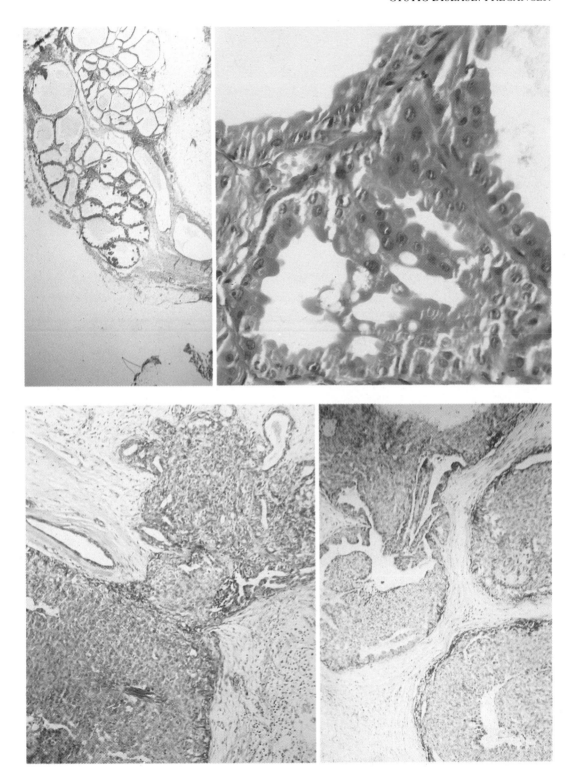

*Fig. 14-3*

*"Blunt duct adenosis"*. This name comes from Foote & Stewart and is not an especially good term for what can be better called hyperplastic lobule. To the left a typical example. The conglomerate of some dilated end tubules constitutes a large lobule, in contrast to the normal lobules seen at bottom right. The hyperplastic lobule has end tubules with rather high papillary epithelium (seen in more detail in the picture on the right). The myothelial layer is very clearly seen.

These hyperplastic lobules are often observed as a part of the ill-defined changes of cystic disease and seem to have no special significance.

*Fig. 14-4*

*Calcifications*. In the breast we often encounter calcifications of different kinds. They have aroused much greater interest since the introduction of mammography. The radiologist sees much more of calcifications than does the histopathologist, who can often find them only after the guidance from radiographs. Calcifications play a very important role in the diagnostics of carcinoma (Sigfusson et al.), although they may also be found in wholly benign or normal conditions.

This picture illustrates "benign" calcifications. To the left and in the center we see many, mostly rounded calcifications varying in size. They are situated in normal or atrophic lobules. They are often concentrically stratified. They are frequently split by the microtome knife or displaced from the section, leaving irregular rifts in the tissue.

To the right, many calcifications lying in connective tissue with no reaction. This is a rare finding which is probably explained by involution of the epithelial elements of lobules.

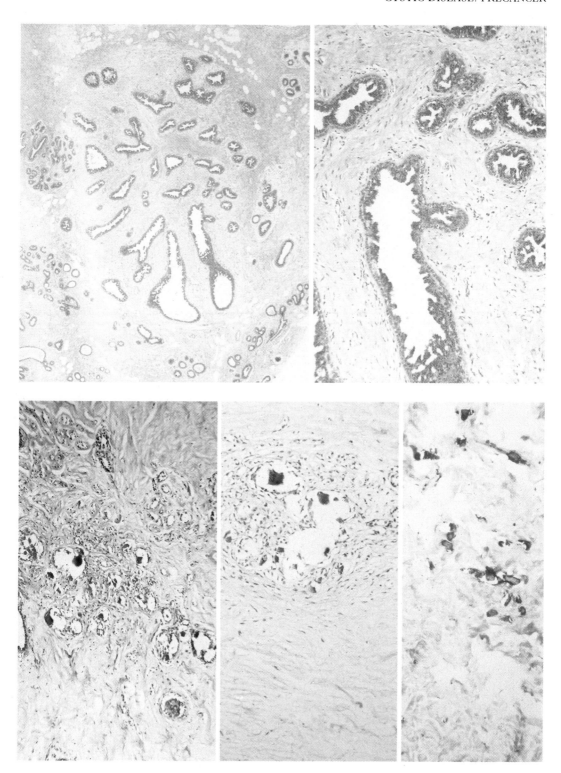

*Fig. 14-5*

*Calcifications.* These are other examples of "benign" calcifications. To the left, some agglomerated dilated ducts with apocrine metaplasia.

In one cyst (arrow) there are numerous calci-spherites. Such calcifications often move when the position of the breast is changed, a phenomenon which signifies benignity.

To the right, a part of a hyalinized fibroadenoma. Even when the epithelium is destroyed we can discern the typical structure (see Ch. 13). In the stroma there are calcifications which have been split by the microtome knife, leaving only splinters along ragged cracks (arrows).

*Fig. 14-6*

*Calcifications in carcinomas.* To the left, a tubular carcinoma. In the lower part, infiltrating small tubules and in the upper part, cribriform intraductal proliferations intermingled with rounded calcispherites.

In the center, essentially the same picture with calcifications in the cribriform intraductal component of a tubular carcinoma.

To the right, an example of the calcification of the type which is most important in the diagnosis of carcinoma. It is an intraductal carcinoma of comedo type with necroses which are calcified (arrow) and split into small pieces.

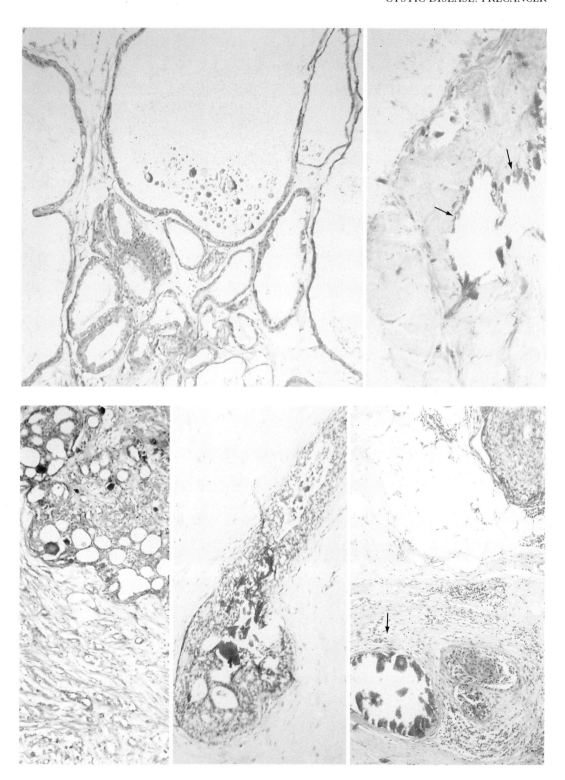

*Fig. 14-7*

*Sclerosing (fibrosing) adenosis*. This name was used by Ewing (1940) to designate an important lesion that has earlier very often been misdiagnosed as carcinoma, and may still be, especially on frozen sections. Its real nature as a proliferation of myoepithelia was early clarified by Hamperl, who did not give the lesion any special name. The lesion is extremely common and will be found in practically all breasts in single or multiple form. These small lesions give no clinical symptoms or macroscopic signs but are incidental findings at microscopy. Then they are mostly confined to one or a few lobules.

The figure shows some such lobules. They consist of an increased amount of tubules, often small and narrow with shallow epithelium. In between there is a proliferation of myothelial cells and some fibroblasts.

There can be rather large variations but the pattern is characteristic. Some variants will be shown in the following pictures.

*Fig. 14-8*

*Sclerosing (fibrosing) adenosis*. Early (?) stage. This picture shows what we imagine to be an early stage. To the left, one rather large lobule, with several separate islands composed of tubules and proliferating myothelia. Several tubules contain calci-spherites, a very common finding in sclerosing adenosis.

This type of change Hamperl called myoepithelial islands, an excellent descriptive name.

To the right, part of the lobule at higher magnification. There is no epithelial atypia. Between the myoepithelial islands there is a loose stroma of the type seen in normal lobules.

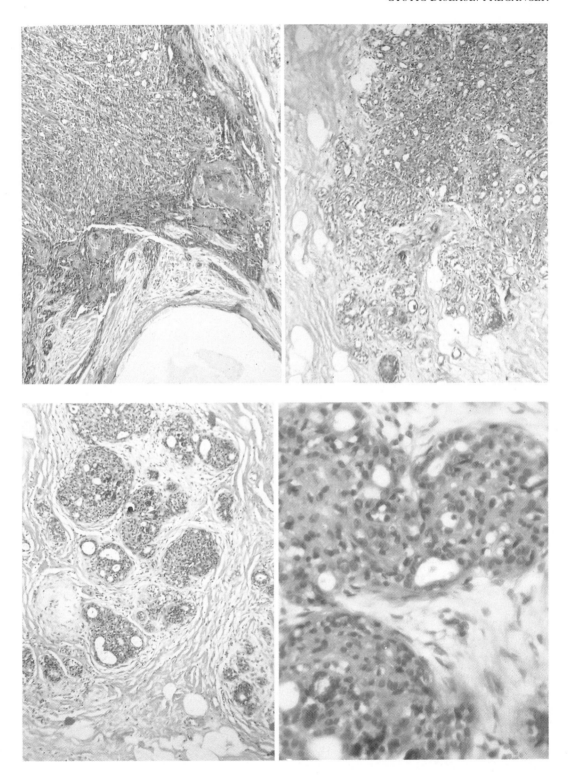

*Fig. 14-9*

*Sclerosing (fibrosing) adenosis.* This is a very characteristic picture. To the left, two lobules, well circumscribed with tightly arranged tubules in a circular pattern. To the right a detail showing tubules with somewhat taller epithelium but without atypia. Mitoses may be seen (arrow) and in some lesions (see Adenosis tumor, Fig. 14-14) they may be numerous.

*Fig. 14-10*

*Myothelial proliferation and invasion of nerves.* Sclerosing adenosis is a benign lesion and statistical studies have failed to provide any evidence that the lesion has any connection with malignant development. This does not exclude the possibility that sclerosing adenosis can be colonized by e.g. lobular carcinoma in situ (Hutter). It has been established for a long time that epithelial elements in sclerosing adenosis can grow into the nerves despite absence of evidence of malignancy. But this is very rare. Sometimes the structure interpreted as a nerve is in reality a normal proliferation of myothelia, cut obliquely.

The picture to the left shows a duct with satellite ducts cut alongside. This quite normal structure can easily be confused with a nerve with epithelial invasion. To the right, a nerve surrounded and invaded (?) by epithelial structures of sclerosing adenosis. It looks more like an embracing of the nerve than a real invasion. Davies (1973) has already pointed out this pitfall (see also Fig. 11-3).

We are convinced that many reported cases are in reality myothelial proliferations around epithelial tubules.

Eusebi & Azzopardi have described vascular invasion in sclerosing adenosis.

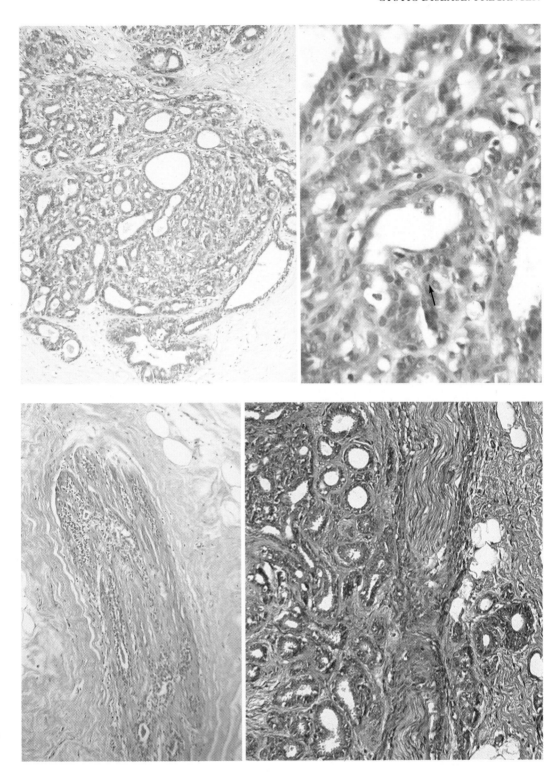

*Fig. 14-11*

*Intraductal sclerosing adenosis (sclerosing intraductal papillomas).* This is an intraductal process that seems to be of essentially the same nature as sclerosing adenosis. Left: In the upper part, ordinary sclerosing adenosis but in the lower part there are two dilated ducts filled with tissue showing sclerosing adenosis (arrows). One of the intraductal proliferations (one arrow) shows central sclerosis and hyalinosis. This structure is shown in the middle. The hyalinization is probably caused by vascular impairment. The tissue around shows narrow tubules in a fibrous tissue with very moderate myothelial proliferation.

Right: An elastin staining showing the elastic tissue in the duct wall.

*Fig. 14-12*

*Intraductal sclerosing adenosis.* This picture is a detail from the left part of the foregoing picture (double arrow). We see a typical picture of sclerosing adenosis with tubules intermingled with myothelial cells. At the arrow there seems to be a budding of the tissue into the duct wall which, however, is preserved around the bud. Probably this is only a branch from the duct filled with the same tissue.

To the right, a higher magnification showing a few tubules and many spindle-shaped myothelial cells.

104

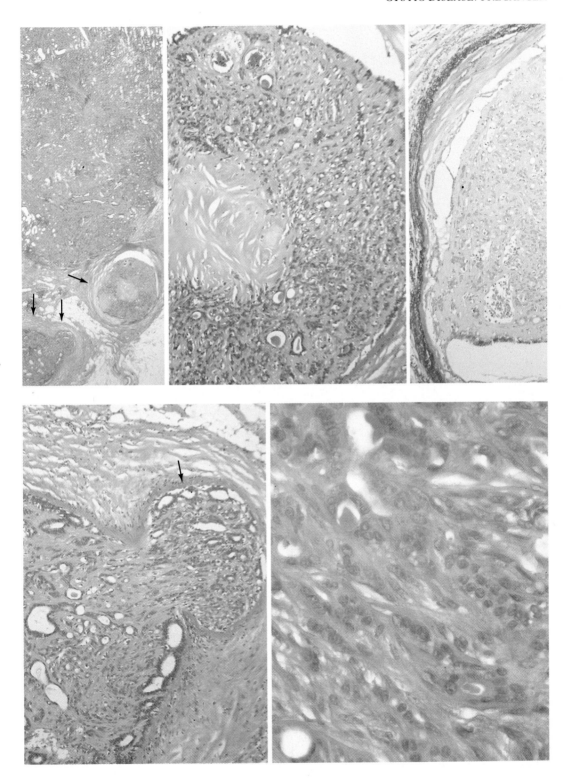

*Fig. 14-13*

*"Ductolobular" sclerosing adenosis*. This is a curious lesion, which is probably a variant of sclerosing adenosis. In the center a branching irregular duct which is embedded in a sharply outlined tissue consisting of myothelial proliferation with remnants of lobular end tubules, some of which are somewhat dilated. The whole lesion may fit under the heading "myoepithelial island".

*Fig. 14-14*

*Adenosis tumor*. This is a type of sclerosing adenosis which is condensed to form a tumor-like lesion. (The name is from Haagensen). It is often seen in young women. By palpation it is hard and may mimic a carcinoma. Even at operation it may be difficult to diagnose. A small piece for frozen section diagnosis has often led to the erroneous diagnosis of carcinoma resulting in ablatio mammae.

Normally we cannot see lobules macroscopically unless they are enlarged as, for instance, in sclerosing adenosis.

The picture to the left illustrates an enlarged lobule. Such large lobules are well delineated, (which is very important for the diagnosis) and mostly rounded. They often appear in clusters. Even at a low magnification the densely packed tubules which constitute the lesion are readily discernible.

To the right, a part of the lobule. The tubules intermingled with myothelial cells are highly differentiated but there can be many mitoses. Apocrine differentiation of the tubular epithelium may also be encountered.

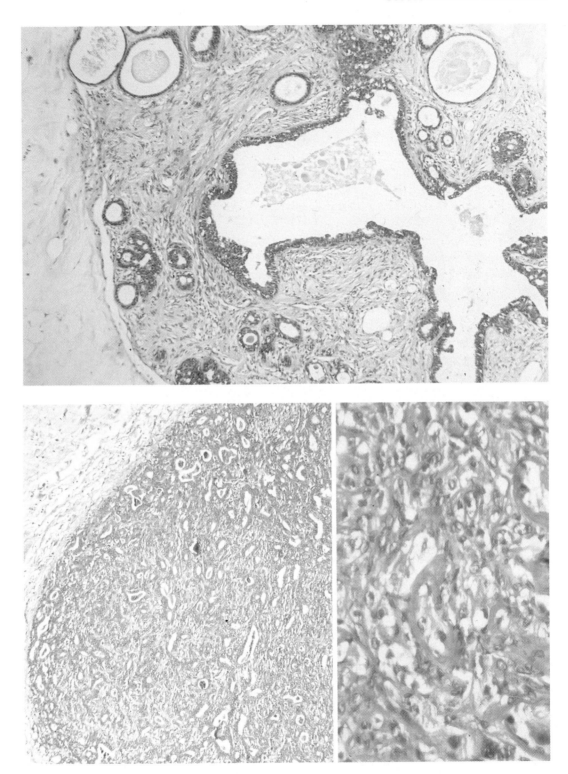

*Fig. 14-15*

*Microglandular adenosis.* This curious lesion is less well known. It seems to have been first described and named by McDivitt & Berg in the tumor atlas of AFIP. However, the type of lesion is not so easily grasped from their two pictures. More detailed descriptions have been given by Rosen (1978 and 1983) and Clement et al. (1983). Rosen has in fact also made the diagnosis in the case presented here. In this case from a 49-year-old woman an ill-defined density was found incidentally in the mammogram. Malignancy was not suspected. The excised specimen was somewhat firm but without clearcut signs of neoplasm.

The lesion is characterized by small tiny tubular proliferations which infiltrate both the fatty tissue and the connective tissue surrounding the lobules. The tubules have shallow, regular epithelium and contain PAS-positive material (see next picture).

The tubules are round and do not have the angulated and drawn out appearance as in tubular carcinoma. As Rosen points out, the tubules are arranged haphazardly and they do not sprout out from a center as is characteristically seen in tubular carcinoma. There are also no elastin deposits. The difference between the normal, more basophilic, lobules is very conspicuous.

*Fig. 14-16*

*Microglandular adenosis.* The same case as in Fig. 14-15. To the left the contrast between the normal lobule and the microglandular structures (arrow). The tubules have shallow epithelium and contain eosinophil material, which is PAS-positive (picture on the right). The lesion may resemble an angioma but the cells have typical epithelial features. The total absence of inflammatory changes is a striking feature as the absence of myothelial cells.

The pathogenesis of this lesion is an enigma. It is said to be rare but when knowledge of the lesion becomes more widespread it will probably be recognized more often. It is probably a benign lesion (Rosen, 1983; Clement et al., 1983).

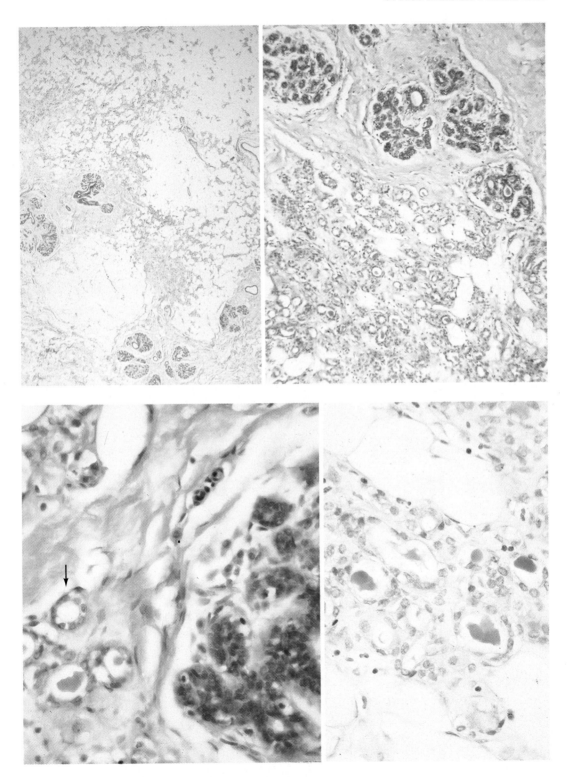

*Fig. 14-17*

*Microglandular adenosis.* This is another case of the same type. A 38-year-old woman with an ill-defined density in the mammogram. The pictures show some normal lobules (arrows) with basophil epithelium. In the connective tissue in between there are irregularly scattered tubules with shallow epithelium. Some of them contained PAS-positive material. The excised specimen contained no fatty tissue. In spite of the infiltration, the tubules appear benign.

*Fig. 14-18*

*Atypical epitheliosis.* In Fig. 14-2 we have shown an example of epitheliosis. In this chapter we will show and discuss some cases of atypical epitheliosis. We have already mentioned that cystic disease with epitheliosis may involve an increased risk of development into carcinoma. It is therefore logical to think that we now and then would occasionally encounter lesions which reside in the borderland between benign and malignant. There is a gray zone between "the white angel" and "the black devil" consisting of lesions without clearcut traits. This zone is very difficult for the diagnosing pathologist, leaving room for subjective views. The following pictures can only illustrate our own views and show examples of cases where we are uncertain and mostly recommend a careful follow-up.

To the left, a duct filled with nearly compact epithelial masses which, however, show clefts lined with regular epithelium. In the lower part, regressive changes with foam cells. In the upper part, outgrowth into a lobule.

To the right, a close-up. The cells are regular and the nuclei are benign looking. Mitoses are few or absent.

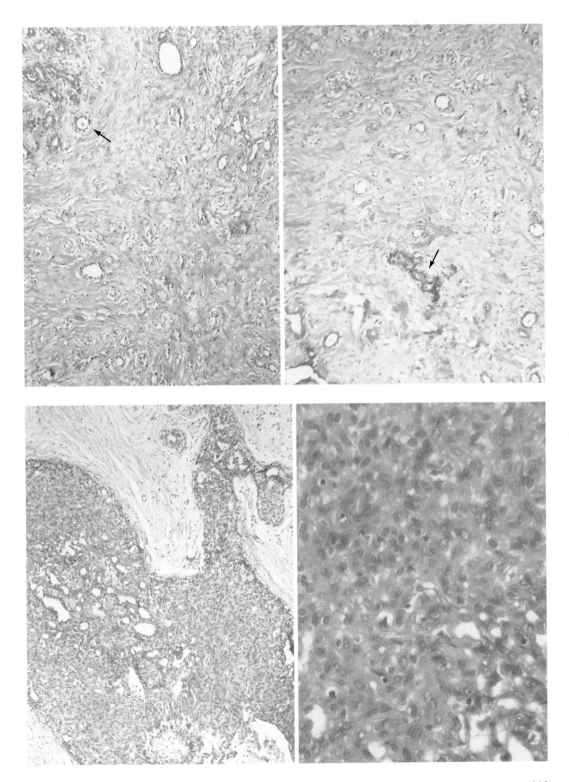

*Fig. 14-19*

*Atypical epitheliosis.* Left: A duct with papillomatous epitheliosis. There is no connective tissue in the stalks. The papillomas are made up of compact epithelial masses but there are clefts and gland-like structures with regular cylindric epithelial cells. There is only very slight cytologic atypia.

Right: Another field form the same case. In the lower part, a papilloma with fibrous stalk, which is considered by many authors to indicate benignity of the lesion (we are not as dogmatic and firm in our faith). In the upper part, the duct has a lining with some slightly atypical micropapillary formations (arrow). Is this the very early beginning of a micropapillary carcinoma? There is no absolute certainty of malignancy but this is clearly a case for close surveillance.

*Fig. 14-20*

*Atypical epitheliosis.* Left: A duct with irregular epithelial proliferations with some cavities filled with foam cells. To the right in the picture there is a part of a small cyst lined by pale apocrine epithelium (arrow).

Right: Another field of the same lesion. In the upper part, epitheliosis in lobules. In the lower part, a cyst lined with slightly atypical bridging apocrine epithelium. There is no certain proof of malignancy. It is our belief that such epithelium can disintegrate and change into foam cells. Probably a process of desquamation will develop, leaving cysts and dilated ducts with detritus.

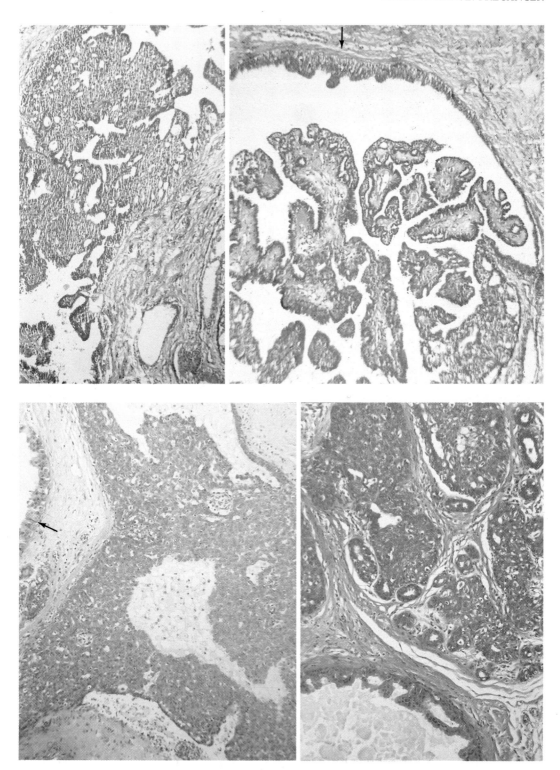

*Fig. 14-21*

*Atypical epitheliosis – intraductal carcinoma?* Two ducts are lined with a highly irregular epithelium, partly shallow, partly multi-layered and papillary. One of the ducts contains cribriform and bridging structures. There is a moderate cellular atypia. To us this lesion arouses a *strong* suspicion of intraductal carcinoma, almost a certain diagnosis. What management should be recommended in a case such as this? This is a matter between the surgeon and the patient after the pathologist has given the surgeon complete information. The therapy may be modified according to the opinion of the patient. In some instances a close control, especially for mammographic calcification, may be justified. In other cases where such a control cannot be performed or the patient insists on having the lesion removed, mastectomy (preferably a subcutaneous one) may be equally justified.

*Fig. 14-22*

*Atypical epitheliosis – intraductal carcinoma?* This is another, similar case. A duct is filled with a blending of cribriform and clustered glandular structures. There is a moderate cellular atypia. Opinions and discussion are much the same as in the foregoing case.

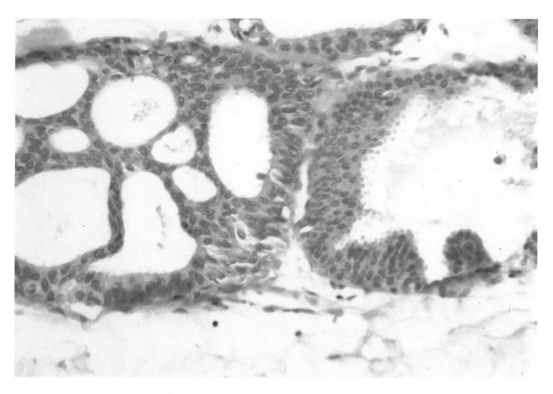

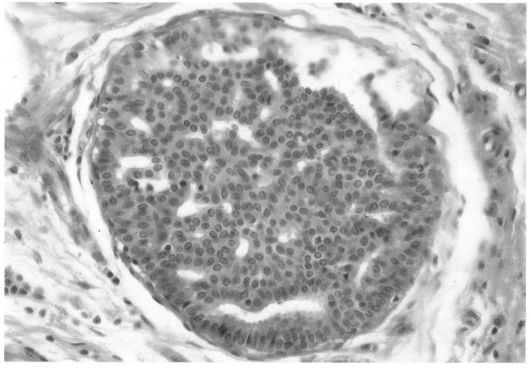

*Fig. 14-23*

*Atypical epitheliosis – early mural carcinoma.* To the left, dilated ducts, lined with epithelium which is clearly atypical. In the small duct there are some papillary projections. They are better seen in detail on the right. Here the irregular epithelium with attempts at bridging and forming papillary projections indicates a mural (clinging) carcinoma. In fact, in other fields there is undisputable mural carcinoma.

*Fig. 14-24*

*Cribriform lobular atypia.* This is a lesion that is very common but less well known. The picture to the left shows some lobules with epithelial hyperplasia. To the right, a high-power field of such lobules. The end tubules of the lobules are dilated and filled with cribriform epithelial proliferations of rather high cyndrical cells. There are often mitoses. This lesion is described by McDivitt et al. in AFIP Atlas under the heading "Atypical terminal duct hyperplasia". These authors believe it to be benign but present no evidence to substantiate this belief. Toker formerly did not distinguish between this lesion and lobular carcinoma in situ but he seems to have separated the two later. We do not know the biologic significance of this lesion. It is very often combined with lobular carcinoma in situ.

Without further knowledge we have no special attitude towards this lesion. Azzopardi depicts such a lesion and says that it is in need of further study. We agree.

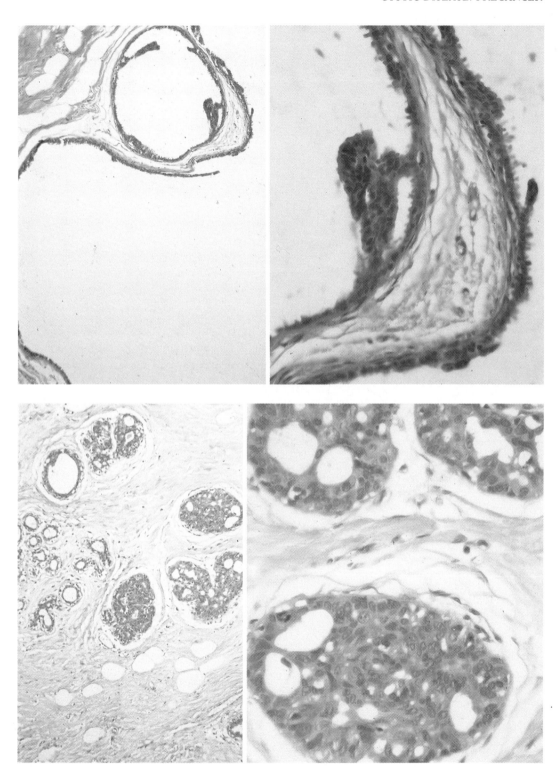

*Fig. 14-25*

*Cribriform lobular atypia.* To the left, a few lobules together with a duct lined by a papillary epithelium. To the right, a detail. Tall, slightly atypical epithelium. At the arrow, a micro-spherolith. We do not know if this change is related to lobular atypia. It may be a vestige of a normal lobule buried in lobular epithelial proliferations.

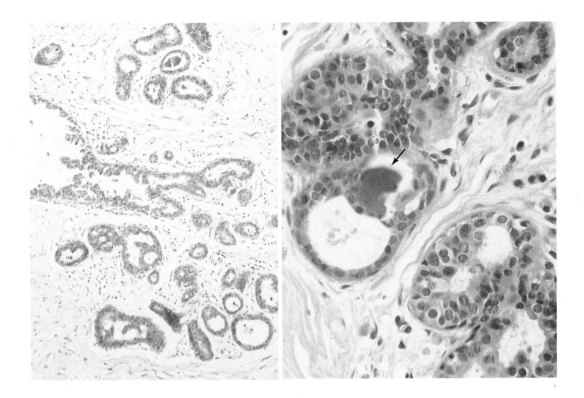

*Fig. 14-26*

*Radial scar.* We use this name for a very characteristic lesion which has previously received little attention. It has been described under various names, viz. proliferation center, rosette (Semb, 1928), sclerosing papillary lesion (Fenoglio & Lattes, 1974), strahlige Narbe (radial scar) (Hamperl, 1975), non-encapsulated sclerosing lesion (Fisher et al., 1979), infiltrating epitheliosis (Azzopardi, 1979), radial scar (Linell et al., 1980). In earlier literature this characteristic lesion was illustrated several times without any special attention being paid to it (for references, see Linell et al., 1980).

Radial scars are very common. Hamperl found 5% in breast biopsies and we found 16% in mastectomies for breast carcinomas. Radial scars are often multiple. We have seen more than 25 in one breast. Most radial scars are very small and cannot be seen with the naked eye, although some are larger, up to 1, or more rarely 2, cm. In mammographies they are sometimes clearly visible as small, spiky lesions, impossible to differentiate from small tubular carcinomas.

The picture shows two radial scars found on mammography. They have an asteroid configuration with radiating grayish-yellow streaks. Macroscopically, they are usually impossible to differentiate from a small carcinoma, though that often feels harder. Sometimes they are combined with small cysts as in the picture to the right.

*Fig. 14-27*

*Radial scar.* The picture shows a rather characteristic example. The center mostly contains abundant elastin deposits, which stain deeply eosinophilic. In most cases (a matter of sampling) one may also find remnants of obliterated ducts often with much elastin in the walls. In the center there are usually haphazardly arranged small tubular structures infiltrating the stroma. This has been described by the meaningless term "pseudoinfiltration".

By definition the tubular structures really infiltrate in the stroma. The word infiltration has a smell of malignancy. The pathologist who judges the tubules to be benign and wants to avoid this word, therefore constructs a new word, "pseudoinfiltration".

Towards the center there is a contraction of surrounding elements of the breast tissue. They consist of fibrous bands containing lobules and ducts in varying proportions. These radiating bands often have a characteristic triangular shape with the apices pointing towards the center (arrows). This orientation suggests that they are formed by contraction towards the center. The architecture of a radial scar is highly characteristic. Although it may show a great deal of variation, which will be illustrated in the following, usually, the general pattern is easily discerned. When one knows what to see, one obtains the ability to see (paraphrase of Goethe).

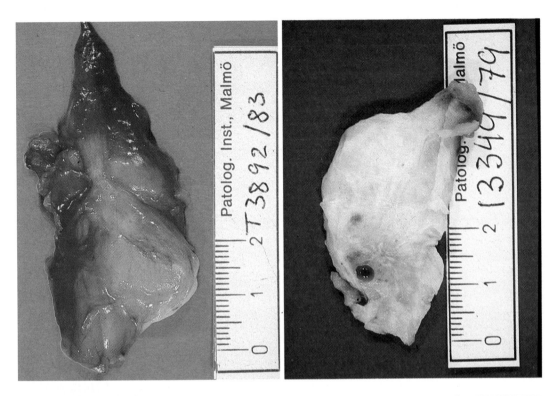

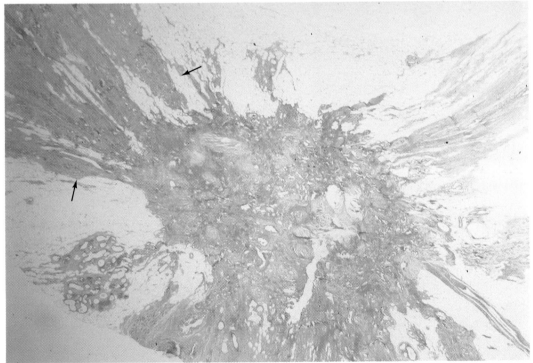

*Fig. 14-28*

*Radial scar.* Two pictures of the same lesion to show the general pattern. To the left, an elastin staining. The center shows elastin deposits, but the infiltrating tubules cannot be discerned in this magnification. The contracted bands contain some small cysts (arrow). In another band there is a group of obliterated ducts (double arrow).

To the right, a silver-staining. The center with elastin deposits is practically free of argyrophil fibers, which are represented in the contracted bands.

In this case the lesion is situated in a part of breast tissue with much fatty tissue. When a scar is situated in breast tissue without fat the retraction bands do not stand out as clearly, but the scar can be recognized by the sclerosed center and the characteristic corona of lobules and ducts contracted around it.

*Fig. 14-29*

*Radial scars.* There are variations in the picture of radial scars but as emphasized earlier there is a common denominator which the experienced histopathologist easily recognizes.

To the left: In the sclerotic center with elastosis there are infiltrating tubules. Contracted against the center is a dilated duct with a papilloma and in the lower part some hyperplastic lobules are oriented against the center.

To the right: A very small radial scar, naturally impossible to see for the naked eye, but in the microscope in a low magnification the general pattern is characteristic. Around the center there is a corona of hyperplastic lobules with tubules, which are somewhat dilated.

122

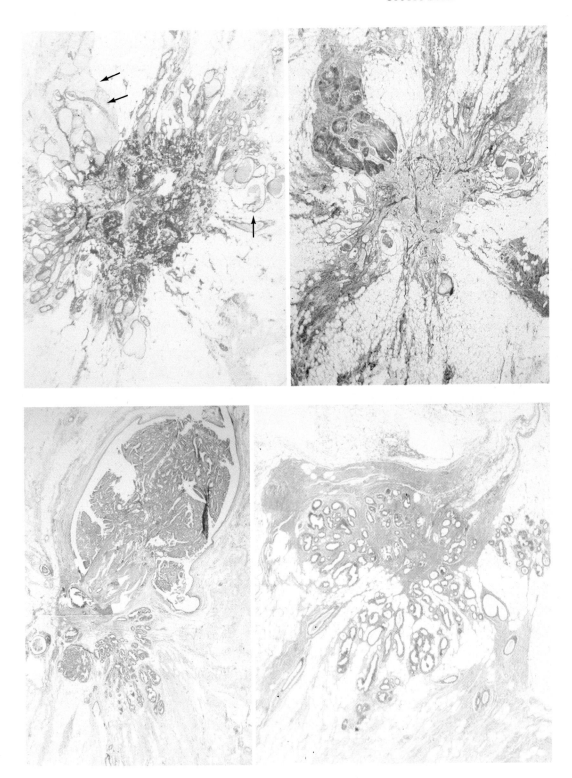

*Fig. 14-30*

*Radial scar.* This scar is somewhat irregular in form. This may partly depend on the orientation of the section. In the center, elastin with partly dilated tubules with shallow epithelium (large arrow). There are at least two obliterated ducts with elastin deposits in the walls (small arrows). The contracted tissue (lower left and upper right) shows lobules with changes of the type seen in cystic breast disease, including small cysts with apocrine epithelium.

The picture of this radial scar may seem atypical, not fitting the general description already given. This is, however, due to the fact that the whole lesion is not included in the picture. A low-power field would have revealed its true nature of being a radial scar with typical architecture.

*Fig. 14-31*

*Radial scar.* Left: Part of radial scar showing essentially the central part. In this an obliterated duct with some remnants of epithelium (see further figs. 14-45-48). Around the center lobules and ducts, some of them with hyperplastic epithelium. In the center also a typical artificial fold.

To the right: A detail of a radial scar with the center showing the "pseudoinfiltration" described in fig. 14-27. The tubules are haphazardly distributed. Some of them have a double cell-layer but often we see tubules without myothelial cells as in the tubules of tubular cancer.

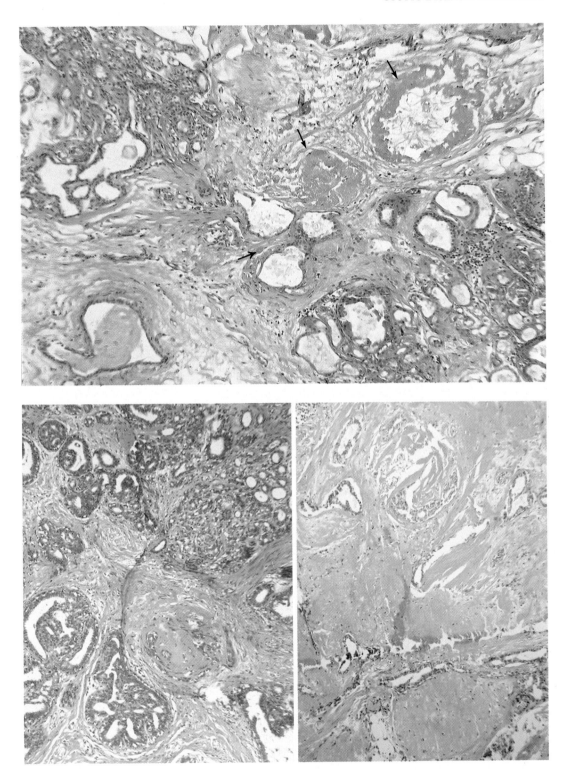

*Fig. 14-32*

*Radial scar.* Two different radial scars to show the variation and, especially, the common basal pattern.

Left: The central part of a radial scar with the center with tubules in a stroma with much elastin (eosinophil). Some of the tubules are dilated which is rather uncommon in the center. Around there are contracted lobules some of which show sclerosing adenosis. This is especially conspicuous in the lower part where the triangular form of the lobule demonstrates the contraction against the center.

Right: The central part of a radial scar with sclerotic stroma rich in elastin deposits. The tubules are distorted and haphazardly arranged.

*Fig. 14-33*

*Radial scar – borderline case.* The two figures show the same part of the center of a radial scar, stained by Htx-eosin and Weigert's elastin staining. The tubules with onelayered epithelium show the same orientation suggesting that they are growing in the same direction against the fatty tissue. Such pictures one often encounters with all types of transitions to the frank infiltration in tubular carcinomas. We therefore call this type borderline case as probably representing the first step in direction of a tubular carcinoma (see the following pictures).

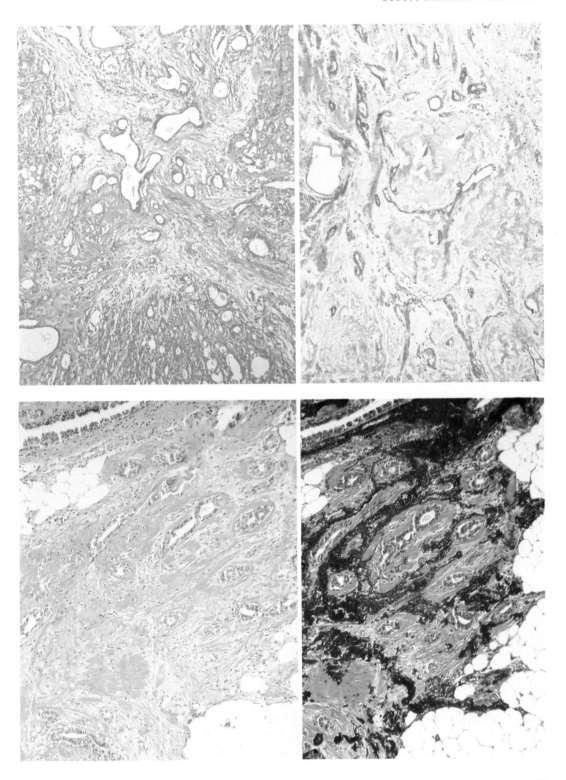

*Fig. 14-34*

*Radial scar – borderline case.* This is a complicated radial scar, difficult to interpret. The upper left shows a general view of the scar, which has its center in the middle of the picture. Above the center and to the right there is a thin-walled cyst. To the left (large arrow) there is a group of ducts, depicted at higher magnification at the bottom left. These ducts have rather tall, slightly atypical epithelium and may represent an intraductal part of a tubular carcinoma. Two arrows point to the area illustrated at higher magnification on the right. A cluster of rather densely packed tubules shows an uneven and ragged border at the fatty tissue and several angulated tubules are (by active growth?) present in the fatty tissue. We also label this case as a radial scar with a strong suspicion of being on its way to becoming a tubular carcinoma.

Hitherto we have maintained a conservative therapeutic attitude in these cases and have recommended radical local excision and close follow-up. We do this with the knowledge that radial scars are often multiple. Many of them probably remain benign. We do not know whether borderline cases always progress to definite tubular carcinomas and the answer to this question is difficult to find.

*Fig. 14-35*

*Radial scar with tubular carcinoma.* This is a very small lesion found incidentally on microscopy of the breast tissue in a case with a carcinoma. An 86-year-old woman with a tubuloductal carcinoma 15×6 mm in size. The lesion was found in a block taken randomly from normal-looking breast tissue.

Left: At the bottom, the center of a radial scar with elastin deposits and an obliterated duct (arrow). In the upper part, a contracted group of cysts, some with rather pronounced papillary epithelial proliferations. In the lower part there are infiltrating tubules on both sides of the obliterated duct and in the high-power microphotograph (picture on the right) we see that it is a clearcut tubular carcinoma infiltrating the fatty tissue with irregular angulated tubules lined with one layer of shallow cells. At the bottom to the right, part of the obliterated duct filled with elastin (arrow).

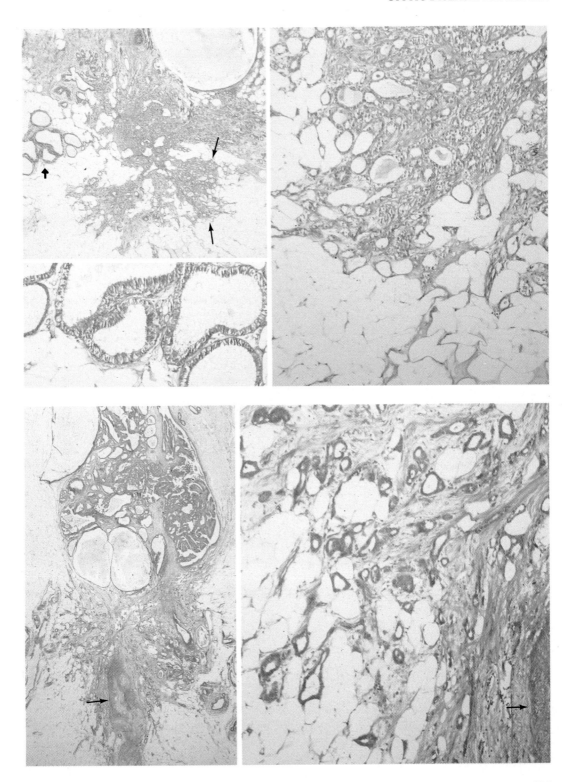

*Fig. 14-36*

*Radial scar with tubular carcinoma*. In a 55-year-old woman screening mammography showed a small spiky lesion. Macroscopically it was a small grayish-yellow star-shaped lesion, reminiscent of a small cancer. It measured 5×4 mm.

Left: Part of a radial scar. At top right is part of the center with much elastin in walls of ducts lined with high epithelium with apocrine snouts. The structure at top right (arrow) is the same as seen at the right of the right hand picture. This shows at high magnification a typical tubular carcinoma growing in the stroma and, on the left side of the picture, out into the fatty tissue. Elastin staining.

*Fig. 14-37*

*Radial scar with tubular carcinoma*. This picture illustrates the importance of adequate sampling. The patient was a 59-year-old woman. At mammographic screening a 10×10 mm large, spiky lesion was found. Two slices from the lesions were embedded.

To the left, part of a radial scar with elastin deposits, sclerotic stroma and very few tubules. To the right, the section from the next slice of the lesion with a tubular carcinoma with ample growth of tubules. Elastin staining.

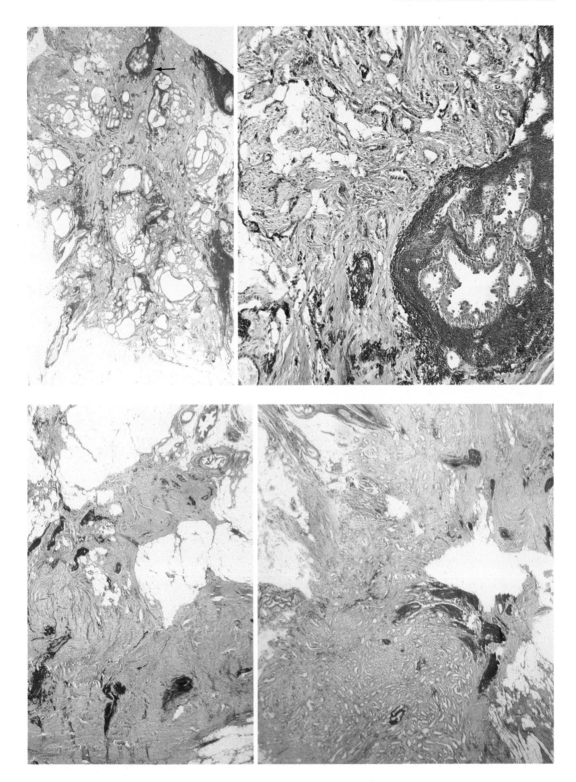

*Fig. 14-38*

*Radial scar with tubular carcinoma.* To the left, elastin stained section of a radial scar. The center shows abundant elastin deposits. Part of the right hand side (arrow) is depicted in the figure on the right, showing a clearcut tubular carcinoma with tubules growing into the fatty tissue.

Hundreds of such cases have convinced us over the years that tubular carcinomas start in radial scars. Fisher et al. made the same observation and described radial scars as "nonencapsulating sclerosing lesions" stating that "these lesions may represent incipient tubular carcinomas".

*Fig. 14-39*

*Radial scar with tubular carcinoma.* At screening mammography of a 44-year-old woman a small spiky lesion measuring 7 mm in diameter was found.

Left: Part of a radial scar with the center at the top with sclerosis and several artificial foldings, mentioned earlier.

At the bottom there are some ducts (arrow). They have an irregular, slightly papillary lining of cells with apocrine snouts. This epithelium may represent the intraductal component of a tubular carcinoma.

Center: What was disclosed from a section of the next slice of the lesion, showing an area where all parts are infiltrated by tubular structures. In the middle the tubules are infiltrating in the rather loose stroma often seen even in tubular carcinomas. But there are also elastin deposits (arrow). Right: Detail of tubules showing lining with epithelial cells with apocrine snouts.

This case also illustrates the importance of adequate sampling in histology.

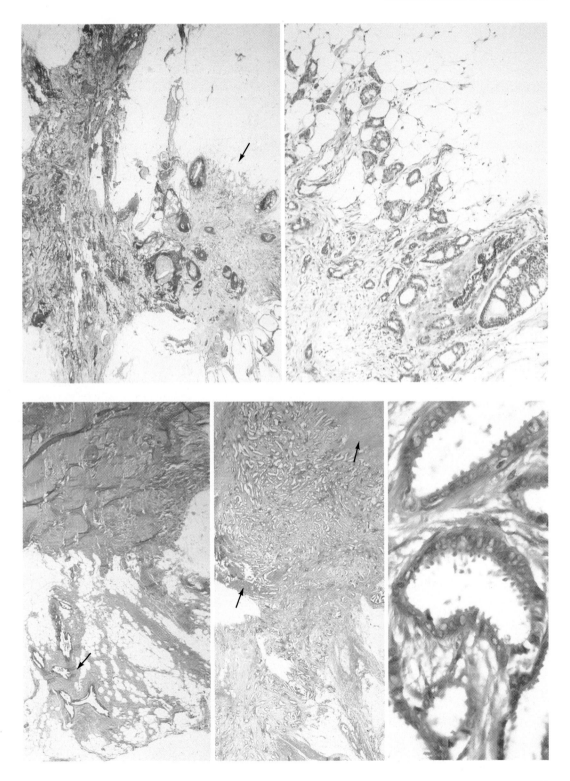

*Fig. 14-40*

*"The smallest tubular carcinoma"*. This is an extremely small radial scar with some dilated ducts in a sclerotic stroma. At one side there is a very small typical tubular carcinoma. To the right one can see the tubules in dense clusters infiltrating the fatty tissue.

*Fig. 14-41*

*Radial scar with tubular carcinoma.* This is also a very early case showing to the left a center of a radial scar with much elastin (eosinophilic). In the sclerotic masses there are haphazardly arranged, narrow, often angulated tubules. To the right, a detail showing the "neoplastic" character of these tubules. They have one-layered epithelium which in some places forms cribriform structures.

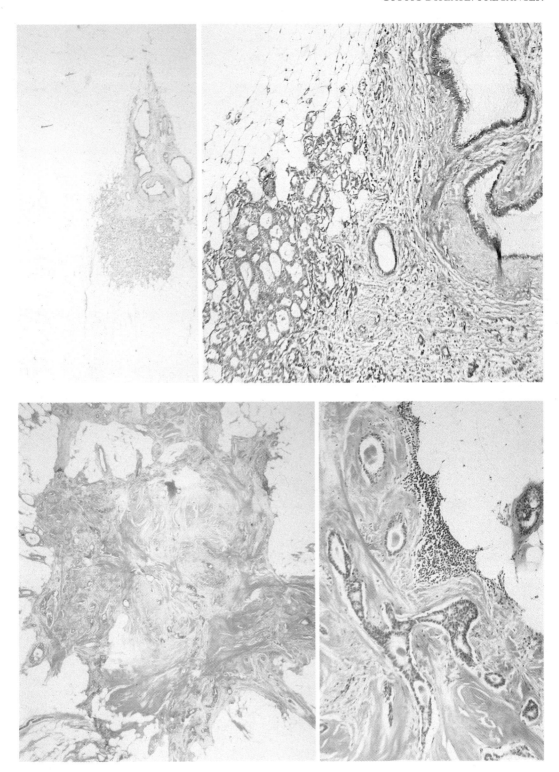

*Fig. 14-42*

*Radial scar with epitheliosis.* This is a typical radial scar with the characteristic artifacts as folds. In this case we have an unusual epitheliosis in the contracted ducts. Epitheliosis in ducts of radial scars is not uncommon but it is uncommon to see as extensive an epitheliosis as here. There is no atypia and no special suspicion of malignancy. But if epitheliosis involves a higher risk of malignancy there is a possibility that a comedo cancer (see further Ch. 15) can start in a radial scar. In reality we see this occasionally, although radial scars are usually the starting points for tubular carcinoma. We have also observed lobular carcinoma in radial scars (see Ch. 15).

A radial scar is undoubtedly related to a duct with surrounding lobules and thus is equivalent to the terminal ductolobular unit, which according to Wellings et al. is the starting point for carcinomas. These authors mostly describe early stages of ductal cancer of comedo type. In their extensive atlas they illustrate two radial scars (Figs. 113-120) and describe them under the heading "miscellaneous compound lesions".

*Fig. 14-43*

*Comedo carcinoma and lobular carcinoma in radial scars.* The origin of ductal carcinoma of comedo type was traced by *Muir* to ducts but Wellings et al. think that the starting point is the lobule. We feel that the latter view is the most probable. In cystic disease one often finds groups of dilated small ducts with apocrine metaplasia. These are obviously derived from lobules. In such groups of lobular ductules we may find all gradations of epitheliosis to frank intraductal carcinoma.

It is quite natural then that a ductal carcinoma of comedo type can also occur in a radial scar.

The left picture shows such a case. There is a typical center of a radial scar with elastosis and infiltrating tubules. Against this center there are contracted lobules and ducts and especially in the left half there is a well developed intraductal carcinoma of comedo type (see further fig. 15-28 and following).

Even lobular carcinoma can be seen in radial scars. To the right part of a radial scar with the center of elastosis down to the left. Around this center there are contracted lobules with end tubules filled with compact masses of small cells (for description of lobular carcinoma see fig. 15-55 and following). They often colonize sclerosing adenosis seen to the lower left.

We are, however, convinced that the type of carcinoma mostly connected with radial scars is the tubuloductal carcinoma as shown in fig. 14-32 and following.

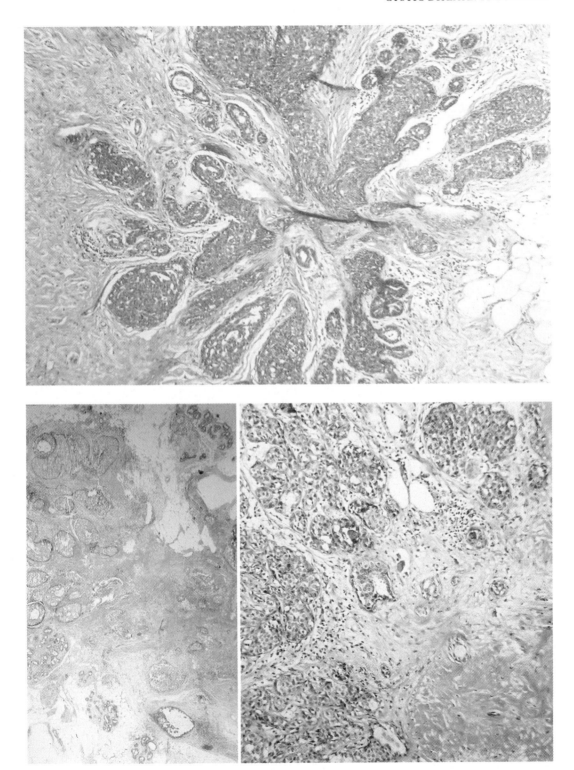

*Fig. 14-44*

*Postoperative scar.* A natural question about the radial scars is how do they develop? Could they result from surgical interventions and other forms of traumatism? After surgery the mammogram may show spiky lesions, although this is rare. These, however, are mostly larger than radial scars. We have never seen lesions after surgery that macro- or microscopically remind us of radial scars. The slides in this case come from a scar with a somewhat streaky appearance, developed after surgery. Microscopically there is no center with elastin as in a genuine radial scar. The contraction in a surgical scar is more diffuse and there are no infiltrating tubules.

*Fig. 14-45*

*Development of radial scars from obliterative duct lesions.* The question from where the radial scars are derived is a very important and interesting one. There is no reason to believe (see the foregoing picture) that they are post-traumatic. The most plausible explanation seems to be the one given by Hamperl (1975) and further corroborated by Egger et al. (1982). The authors believed that they develop through shrinkage in "mastopathia obliterans" known for a long time and regarded as the end result of retention syndrome. Such obliterating lesions are depicted in Ch. 12. The epithelial remnants from satellite ducts may be the forerunners of the infiltrating tubules in the radial scar centers.

Left: A detail from a center of a radial scar with large elastin masses. The small tubules with one-leyered, shallow epithelium could well be epithelial remnants of satellite ducts.

This will be even more evident in the following pictures. This picture shows a small radial scar. In the center there is an obliterated duct (arrow) with an easily discernible contour. This duct is shown at higher magnification in the next picture.

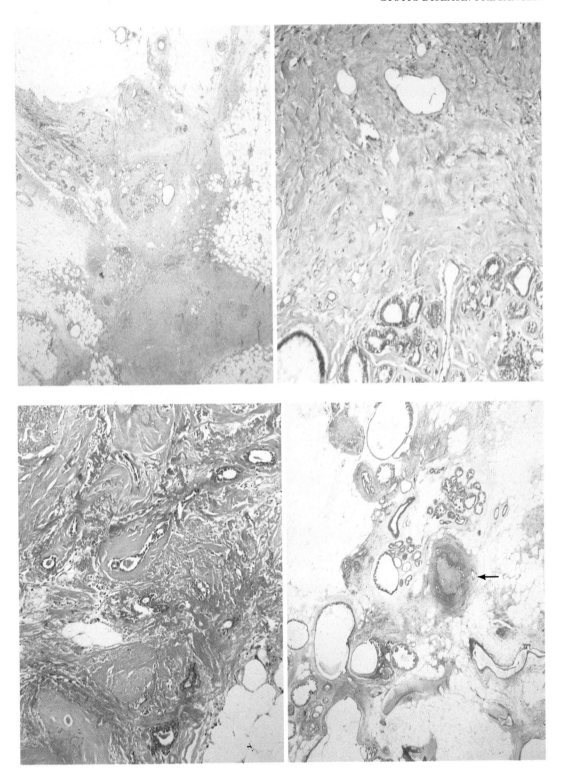

*Fig. 14-46*

*Development of radial scars from obliterative mastopathies.* These are details of the obliterated duct seen in the foregoing picture. It is replaced by a mass of hyalinized connective tissue surrounded by small ducts. These small ducts may be remnants of satellite ducts. To the right we see the same in Weigert's elastin staining. There are abundant elastin masses in the outer parts of the obliterated duct, probably representing the connective tissue mantle of the duct wall.

Pictures of this type are often seen and have been illustrated by Hamperl (1975) and Linell et al. (1980). In the latter book are also discussed the many avenues of research that open up when it is realized that as many as half of all breast carcinomas may begin in radial scars. If these are consequences of obliterating mastopathies they may well be related to hormonal influences, desquamative processes, etc., which, in turn, may be related to different risk groups such as nulliparous or late parous women.

*Fig. 14-47*

*Obliterative mastopathies.* This is a rather common picture. A duct is totally obliterated by granulation tissue. This often contains fat-laden macrophages. The preservation of epithelial elements, obviously derived from the satellite ducts, is characteristic. The cause of obliteration is probably in many cases secretion stagnation and the debris will later be organized by granulation tissue. These changes have been collectively designated the "retention syndrome", which has been more fully discussed in Ch. 3 and 12. A further stage in these events may be the formation of a radial scar (see the following picture).

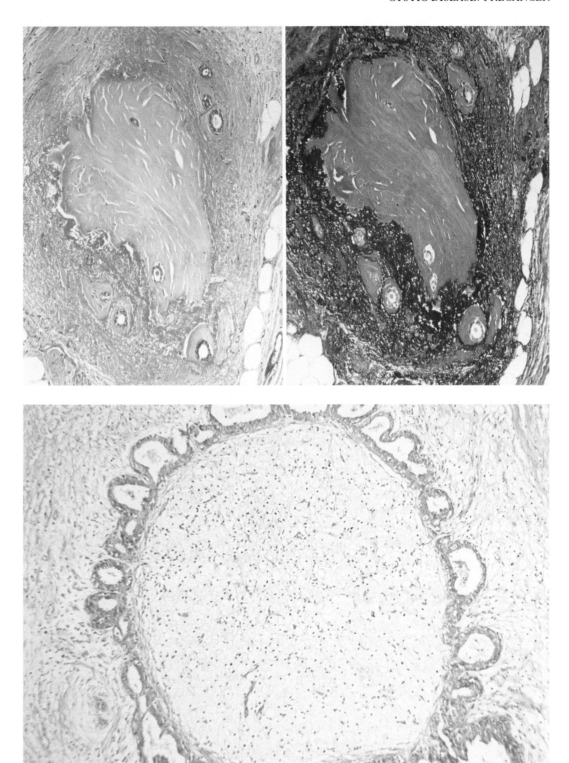

*Fig. 14-48*

*Obliterative mastopathy developing into radial scar.* To the left an incipient radial scar. Several ducts and lobules are oriented in a fashion, pointing to retraction towards a center (arrow), characterized by eosinophil masses of elastin containing a small rounded structure. This is more clearly seen to the right. It is obviously an obliterated duct and in the periphery there is a ring of small tubules with one-layered epithelium. The sequence from obliterative mastopathy to radial scar seems to be well established.

*Fig. 14-49*

*"Radial scar" in lung tissue.* Already in the forties Roessle and collaborators had put forward the conception that many carcinomas start in scars in the lung tissue. This idea was later elaborated and confirmed by Meyer & Liebow (1965). As illustration we show a case of "radial scar" in the lung, found incidentally on microscopy of a randomly taken lung piece at autopsy (arrow). The scar looks like the center of a radial scar with abundant elastin and a few, small, epithelium-lined slits. There is an evident contraction of the surrounding tissue towards the center.

It may be possible to find a relationship between scarring and carcinomas in other organs, e.g. the papillary carcinomas of the thyroid, which sometimes have sclerotic centers with abundant elastin deposits.

The more intimate mechanism in cancerogenesis is unknown but we refer to theories about the complicated interactions of carcinogenic factors with stroma and epithelium (for references, see Petri, 1979).

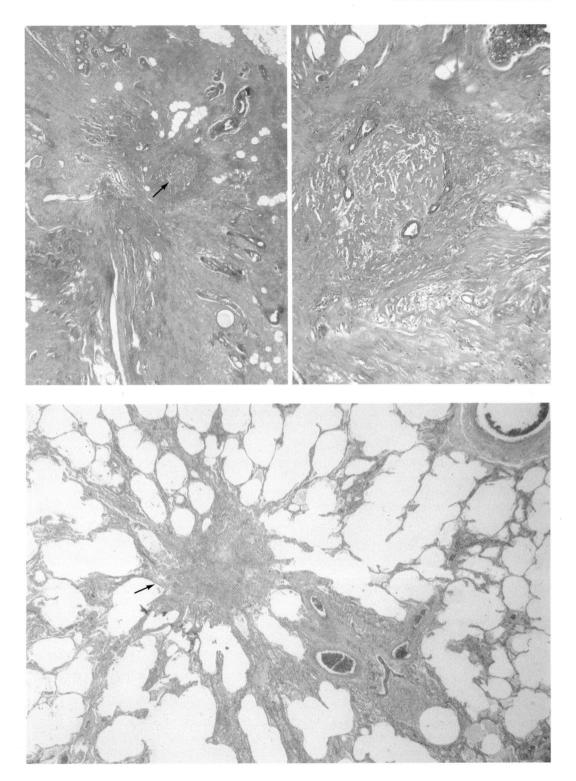

# Chapter 15

# Carcinomas

*Fig. 15-1*

*Tubular carcinoma.* Tubular carcinoma was formerly almost unknown and thought to be very rare. Nowadays, as reported in chapter 6., it is a common finding, especially in screening material. Against this background was conceived the idea of their development from radial scars and their further progression to less differentiated tubuloductal carcinomas (see Ch. 14 and Ch. 15). In older material tubular carcinoma or well differentiated adenocarcinoma (the name used by Taylor & Norris) only constituted 1-2%; the frequency now is about 10 times higher. Tubular carcinomas are easy to find by mammography because retractions are easily seen (Linell et al., 1980).

Macroscopically, tubular carcinomas are mostly small (often less than 1 cm). They are hard and have a stellate appearance with gray-yellow streaks of elastin. In the left picture the tumor is situated at the border of the parenchymal disc and retractions in the fatty tissue can be seen in the upper part. To the right, a small stellate tumor situated in adipose tissue.

Due to its radial appearance, tubular carcinoma is usually easy to recognize in the mammogram but when the same lesion, after local excision, is examined by specimen radiography, it is often found to have lost its spiculated appearance. This illustrates that the spicules (retractions) are not stiff cancerous outgrowths, but connective tissue bands which, when cut off during the excision of the tissue, lose their anchorage in the surrounding tissue whereby the tumor assumes a more rounded shape.

*Fig. 15-2*

*Tubular carcinoma.* This is an extremely small tubular carcinoma found incidentally on histologic study of a breast operated on for other indications. Left: A view of the whole lesion with sclerosis and elastin deposits in the lower part. In the central part there are some ducts with cribriform growth. Tubular carcinoma is often combined with intraductal carcinoma (65% according to Carstens). Such figures are of relatively little use because they are highly dependent on the sampling of material for histology. In our opinion the intraductal component is an integral part of tubular carcinoma. At the upper right, the carcinoma infiltrating the fatty tissue. Right: This infiltration of tubules at higher magnification.

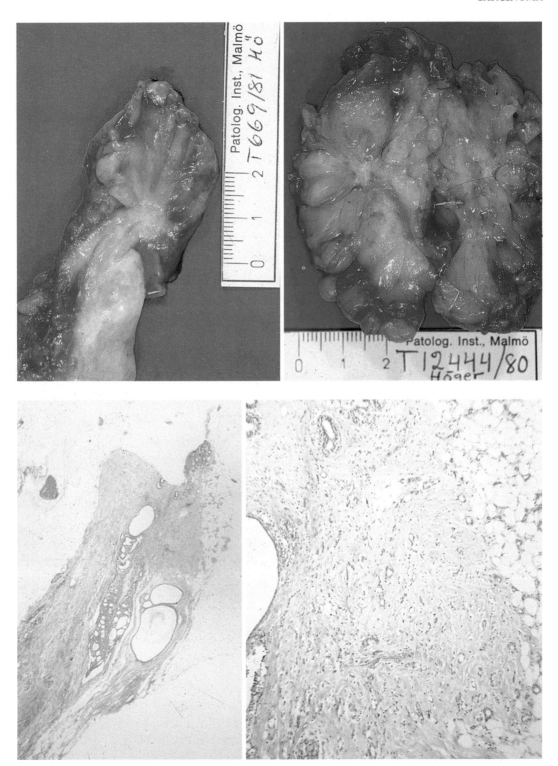

*Fig. 15-3*

*Tubular carcinoma.* This is a small stellate tumor with many spicules. These spicules are retractions of tissue from the surroundings towards the center. They contain connective tissue with lobules and ducts. In one of the spicules there is a small cystic duct with conspicuous elastin in the wall (arrow). The carcinoma can grow out into the spicules (double arrow) but mostly it grows between them, giving the tumor a more even and rounded contour (three arrows) (see Linell et al., 1980). The abundant elastin deposits are clearly seen as eosinophil masses to the left in the hematoxylin-staining. To the right, the same deposits in Weigert's elastin-staining. The infiltrating carcinoma can be dimly seen as a delicate lace-work in the periphery of the tumor (three arrows).

*Fig. 15-4*

*Tubular carcinoma.* Left: A picture of the central part. At upper left, a thick-walled duct with preserved epithelial lining. The large eosinophil masses are elastin deposits in thick-walled ducts, some of which are wholly obliterated. In between the thick-walled ducts there is a looser stroma with infiltrating tubules. Right: These tubules in a loose cellular stroma. The tubules are irregular and angulated, and haphazardly dispersed. The tubules have one-layered, rather shallow epithelium. There is very little atypia and mitoses are very rare.

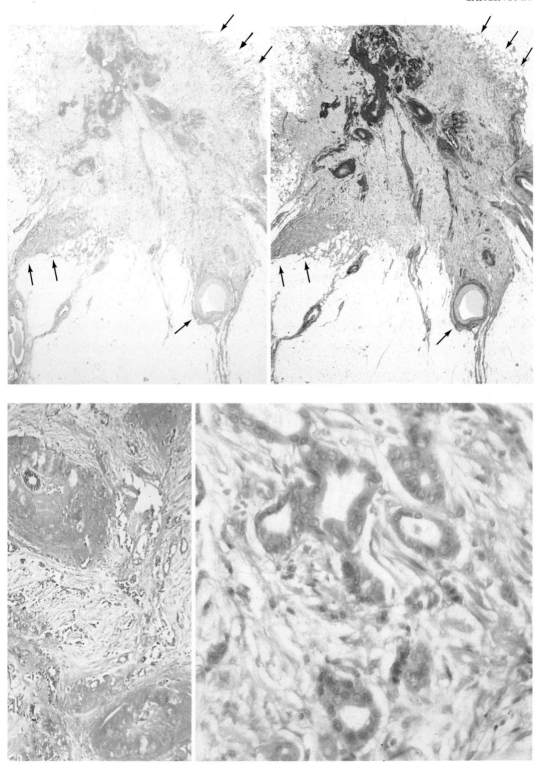

*Fig. 15-5*

*Tubular carcinoma.* Another example to show the variations. Left: A small part of a tubular carcinoma. In the upper part, the border of the tumor with lymphoid infiltrates partly forming lymphoid follicles. Such lymphoid infiltration is seldom seen in tubular carcinomas. The lower part shows the carcinoma, which in this case is dominated by the cellular stroma, a characteristic feature in some cases of tubular carcinoma.

Right: The cellular stroma with haphazardly arranged, narrow, angulated, infiltrating tubules. At lower right, a cribriform intraductal growth of carcinoma. From some recent reports on tubular carcinoma one gets the impression that the authors look upon the intraductal carcinoma as an coincidental finding in tubular carcinoma. We feel, however, that both intraductal and infiltrating components are integral parts of tubular carcinoma.

*Fig. 15-6*

*Tubular carcinoma.* Left: An intraductal cribriform carcinoma in a thin-walled duct. In the surrounding stroma there are abundant elastin deposits. This type of intraductal growth is highly characteristic of tubular carcinomas. It can be seen centrally in the tumor and also in the surroundings of the infiltrating carcinoma. The diagnosis tubular carcinoma is rarely made without infiltrating tubules. We are convinced that purely intraductal cases of tubular carcinoma exist. In such cases the intraductal component must have the characteristic appearance seen here to the right. In Ch. 14 is another example. Compare also Fig. 15-7.

Right: An infiltrating tubular carcinoma, seen at lower right. At upper left, a thick-walled tortuous duct with tubular and cribriform carcinoma growing in connective tissue, filling the duct. In one place (arrow) there is a breakthrough of these structures out into the stroma, demonstrating the connection between intraductal and infiltrating components.

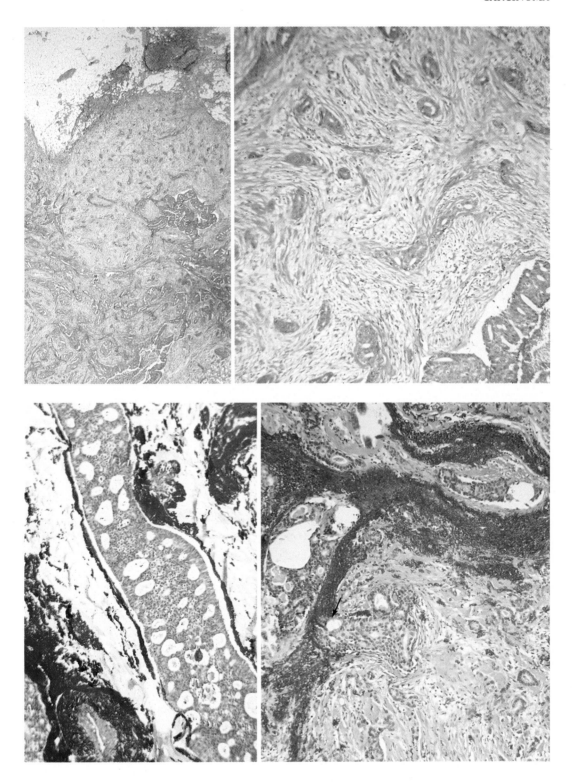

*Fig. 15-7*

*Tubular carcinoma. Intraductal component with microliths.* A higher magnification of intraductal cribriform carcinoma in tubular carcinoma. Moderate atypia. Several laminated microliths are seen. In the lower part of the picture some cells have apocrine snouts (arrow), a common finding in tubular carcinoma.

Calcifications of the type shown here are very common findings in tubular carcinomas. However, calcifications are not of the same diagnostic value in mammography as in comedo carcinoma (see Figs. Ch. 13) because tubular carcinoma has other, more significant, features, i.e. stellate structure with retractions. Naturally, calcifications are a supplementary support in the mammographic diagnosis.

*Fig. 15-8*

*Tubular carcinoma with a minor component of compact "ductal" structures (tubular carcinoma +++).* Already in earlier descriptions (Taylor & Norris, 1970) it is pointed out that many tubular carcinomas are not pure but also contain more undifferentiated compact "ductal" strands. In reality more than 50% of what are called tubular carcinomas contain parts of those less differentiated structures. In our opinion this is an expression of tumor progression towards less differentiated, more aggressive tumor types. This is only the first step in progression described elsewhere (Ch. 6 and Ch. 15).

To the left, the central part of such a tumor. In the upper field, intraductal cribriform growth (note the "apocrine snouts" of the cells). In the lower part, infiltrating tubules.

To the right the peripheral border of this tumor with few tubules and mostly less differentiated compact "ductal" structures. Such changes can be seen in the whole periphery or in only a small part of it.

Most papers about tubular carcinomas include both pure tubular carcinomas (Tub. ca. ++++) and cases with a minor part of less differentiated "ductal" elements (Tub. ca. +++). These two types are mostly summarized as tubular carcinoma (well differentiated adenocarcinoma).

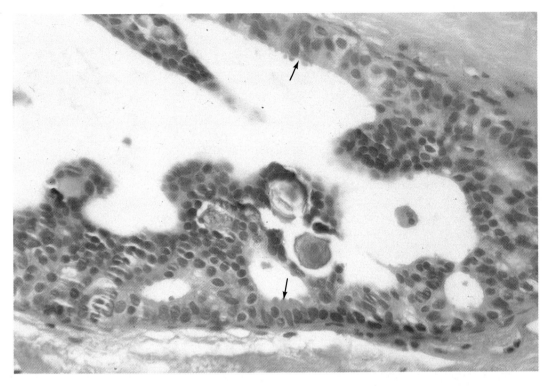

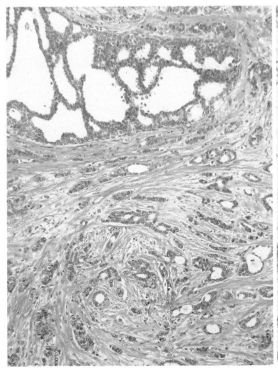

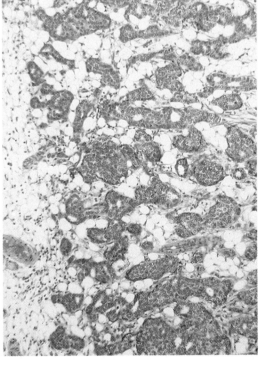

*Fig. 15-9*

*Tubular carcinoma (Remnants of radial scars).* Not in the first but in rather early descriptions it was pointed out that abundant elastin deposits was a typical feature of tubular carcinomas. There is now ample evidence that they represent remnants of radial scar (see Ch. 5, Ch. 6 and Ch. 14).

To the left, the central part of a tubular carcinoma with thick-walled, obliterated ducts with elastin in the walls. There are infiltrating tubules around them.

To the right, another example of the central part of a tubular carcinoma. In the upper part, an obliterated duct where the lumen is filled with a rather loose connective tissue. In the picture there are no tubules. The importance of an adequate sampling of such lesions has already been emphasized (Ch. 14).

In our study of about 500 carcinomas (Linell et al., 1980) we found that about half of infiltrating carcinomas showed signs that could be interpreted as remnants of earlier radial scars. Fisher et al. (1983) in a large study of 1600 cases found remnants of scars in about ⅓ of the cases. Considering possible differences in carcinoma materials (Ch. 6) there are reasons to believe that our results are in good agreement.

*Fig. 15-10*

*Metastasis of tubular carcinoma.* It was formerly said that metastases from tubular carcinoma were seldom seen. This is wrong. In our material about 10% of pure tubular carcinomas have metastasized. The figure shows a metastasis from a tubular carcinoma + + +. As often seen the metastasis is purely tubular (Linell et. al. 1980). It has also been claimed that when tubular carcinoma metastasizes, this is often confined to the lowest node in the axilla. We cannot confirm this. We often find metastases higher up in the axilla. Another observation is that the metastases often show periglandular growth (see next picture).

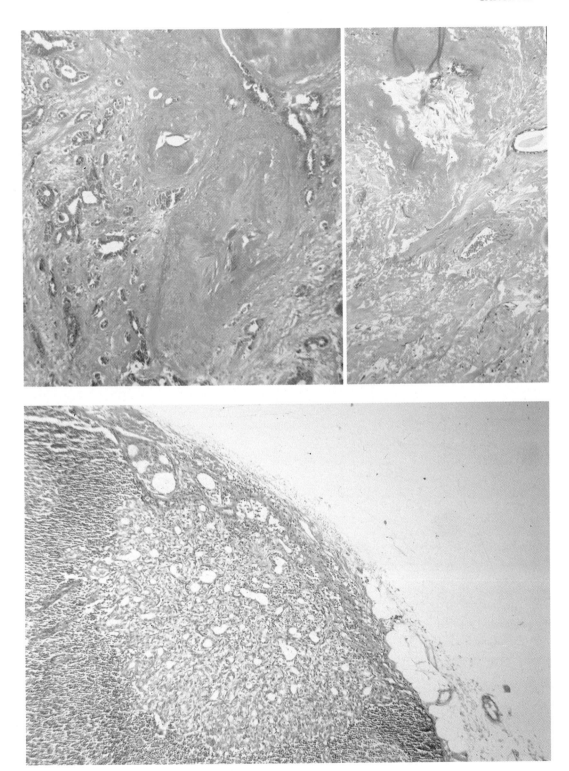

*Fig. 15-11*

*Metastasis of tubular carcinoma.* Metastases from tubular carcinomas are often small and marginal but nevertheless they often grow through the capsule and show perinodal growth. We are not convinced that perinodal growth always denotes a bad prognosis.

To the left, a small lymph node. The capsule in the upper part seems to be thickened; as will be seen later, this is due to a small marginal metastasis. Outside this part of the lymp node there are many fibrous strands.

To the right, at higher magnification, it is evident that this represents a marginal metastasis with growth through the capsule and widespread growth in the surroundings.

This type of growth is seen very often in small lymph nodes. Other carcinomas, e.g. comedo carcinoma, often have large lymph node metastases, though frequently without perinodal growth.

*Fig. 15-12*

*Tubular carcinoma. Elastin deposits in metastasis.* There has been much discussion about the production of elastin. It is extremely interesting to study the deposition of elastin in metastasis of tubular carcinoma. Azzopardi has pointed to the frequent elastosis in metastatic deposits of breast carcinoma, even in such localities as pancreas and gut.

To the left, a marginal metastasis of a tubular carcinoma. There is growth of tubules in the capsule and in the surroundings and eosinophil deposits (arrows) can be seen. At the upper right, elastin stained deposits in close connection with the tubules. This speaks for the ability of the infiltrating tubules from tubular carcinoma to induce deposition of elastin. It may be speculated whether the same phenomenon may occur in the elastin-rich centers of radial scars (see Ch. 14).

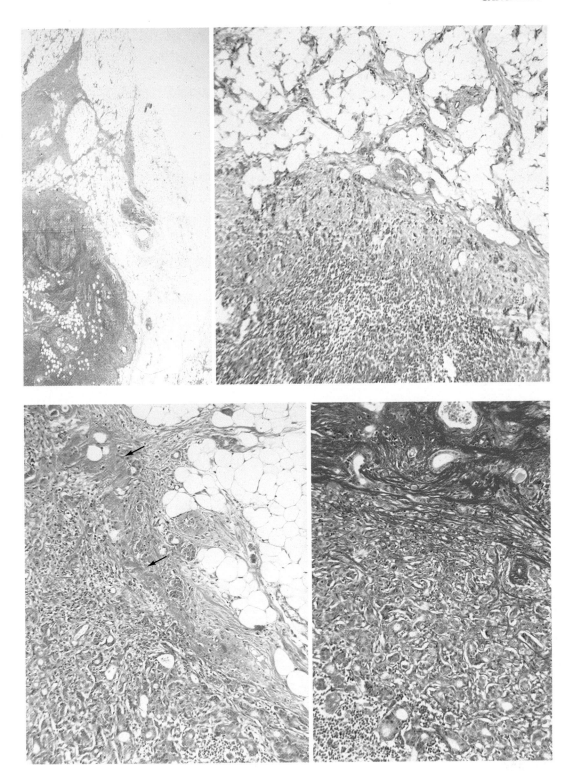

*Fig. 15-13*

*Tubuloductal carcinoma (Invasive ductal carcinoma).* In Ch. 6 tubuloductal carcinoma was classified as a special group. This group may well correspond to "duct carcinoma with productive fibrosis" (Foote & Stewart) or "stellate carcinoma" (Azzopardi) but has been lost in the big group "duct carcinoma N.O.S." (not otherwise specified) of Saphir, Fisher, or Rosen. These tumors have a very characteristic macroscopic appearance. They are mostly very spiculated, extremely hard and show typical gray-yellow streaks, which are not necroses as formerly believed but deposits of elastin in duct walls or diffusely in the stroma. These tumors often show the typical orange-yellow border (see Fig. 15-27). This is nearly pathognomonic for this type of tumor but is rarely seen in other carcinomas. In Ch. 6 we have divided this group into three subtypes, tubular carcinoma + +, + and 0, according to the proportion of tubular structures. This was hypothetically interpreted as a result of a continuous or discontinuous *progression* of tubular carcinomas towards less differentiated stages. From the beginning this had a purely histologic basis, but has later on been statistically substantiated by the good correlation found with the size of the tumors (Ch. 6) and with the number of lymph node metastases (Ch. 6). The histologic picture of metastases speaks also for a progression from highly to less differentiated forms. So does the mammographic picture (Linell et al., 1980) as well, showing a change in shape of the tumors from a highly stellate to a more rounded appearance with decreasing degree of differentiation.

To the left, a small spiculated tumor. Due to contraction the cut surface of the tumor looks depressed. The tumor shows grayish-yellow streaks. This tumor was histologically characterized as tubular carcinoma + +.

To the right, a slightly larger tumor, showing essentially the same macroscopic picture. This spiculated star-shaped tumor showed, as even small tumors of this type do, the typical "pinching" of the skin which is caused by a traction of surrounding structures and not by cancerous outgrowth.

*Fig. 15-14*

*Tubuloductal carcinoma (tubular carcinoma + +) (Invasive ductal carcinoma).* Left: Central part of the tumor. Tubules with low regular epithelium growing in a loose fibroblastic stroma with much elastin deposits. The ancestry of a "tubular carcinoma" is very suggestive.

Right: Periphery of the same tumor. The infiltration into the fatty tissue consists of less differentiated "ductal" structures. The cells are regular with few mitoses. "Cancerization of lobules", so often found in ductal carcinoma of comedo type, is practically never seen in tubuloductal carcinomas.

It is easy to see that on the whole this tumor shows the same characteristics as some tubular carcinomas (for instance fig. 15-8 tubular carcinoma + + +). It seems natural to interpret them as expressions of different stages in a progression. At the same time it is obvious that comedo carcinoma behaves different. Unfortunately, in most other classifications these two types are grouped together as ductal carcinoma (N.O.S.).

In a recent paper (Fisher et al., 1983) the carcinomas are divided into two large groups, which seem to correspond very well to our groups. They call them "scar-cancers" and "non-scar cancers".

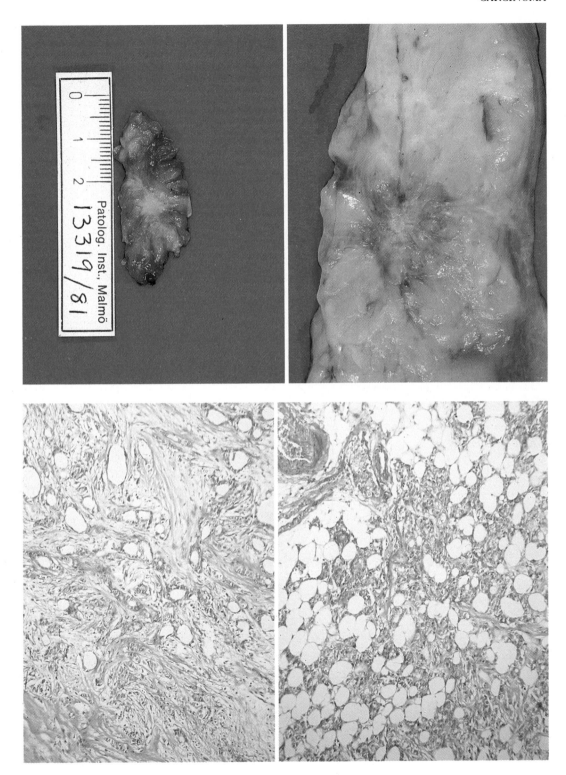

*Fig. 15-15*

*Metastasis from a tubuloductal carcinoma (Invasive ductal carcinoma).* The metastasis is a mixture of "ductal" and tubular structures, the latter dominating. Even in tumors progressing towards a less differentiated component one can find many tubules in the metastases. We do not know whether this is an expression of "differentiation" in the metastasis or an indication of the metastasis having been already established when the primary tumor had not yet progressed to a lesser differentiated stage.

There is a continuous shift from tubular structures in the lymph node metastases towards "ductal" or compact cancer strands.

The findings in a rather large series of metastases are tabulated in Linell et al. (1980).

*Fig. 15-16*

*Tubuloductal carcinoma (tubular carcinoma + +)(Invasive ductal carcinoma).* This is a small, spiculated tumor. In the central part there are moderate to rich deposits of elastin. Elastin deposits in varying amounts are always seen in tubuloductal carcinomas if the sampling is adequate. It should be realized that if only one section is made and it happens to cut in the periphery, elastin may be scanty or absent. The following picture shows details of this tumor.

This is a typical example of a "stellate" tumor. The center is rather sclerotic and the periphery more "medullary". One can also see that the cancerous growth into the fatty tissue (arrow) is preferably located between the spicules, giving the tumor a more rounded shape. Elastin stain.

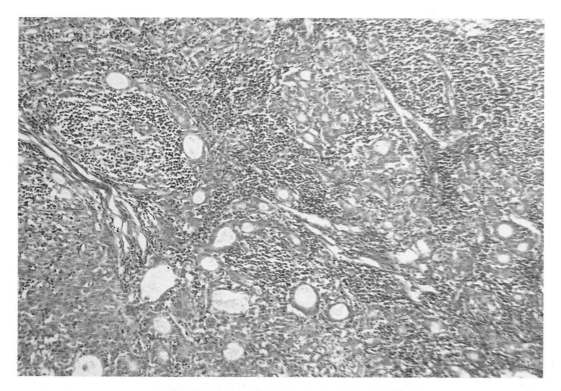

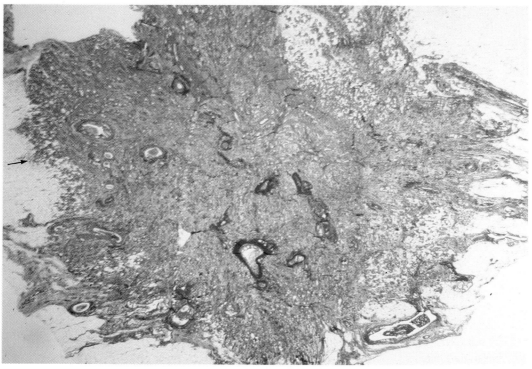

*Fig. 15-17*

*Tubuloductal carcinoma (tubular carcinoma + +) (Invasive ductal carcinoma).* This is the same tumor as in Fig. 15-16.

Left: Central part of the tumor. Two ducts show intraductal cribriform carcinoma and around them infiltrating tubules with shallow epithelium. The eosinophil masses in the stroma are elastin deposits.

Right: Periphery of the tumor with less differentiated "ductal" columns. The cells are rather regular. There is no cancerization of lobules. A few tubules are seen. The cells in the periphery of the columns are darker, which has been suggested to be an expression of metabolic change in RNA-metabolism (Caspersson & Santesson). This is a general feature found in all cancer columns and probably due to better nutrition in the periphery of the cancer column than in the more central parts lying further away from the vessels.

*Fig. 15-18*

*Tubuloductal carcinoma (tubular carcinoma +) (Invasive ductal carcinoma).* This is another example of tubuloductal carcinoma to show the supposed progression. The difference from the foregoing case may seem rather small.

The central part shows abundant elastin deposits both in duct walls and diffusely in the stroma. The epithelial structures in this part are mostly tubular. To the right (arrows) we see outgrowth of undifferentiated, "ductal", solid columns of carcinoma cells. Elastin stain.

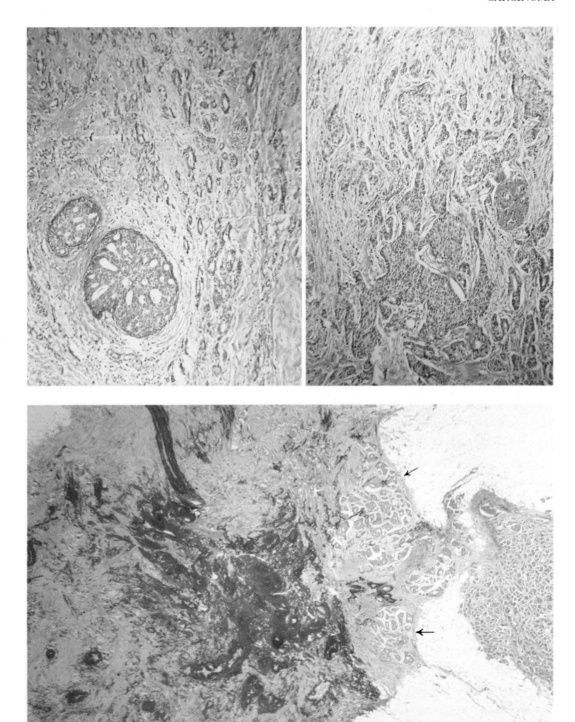

*Fig. 15-19*

*Tubuloductal carcinoma (tubular carcinoma +) (Invasive ductal carcinoma).* The pictures are details of Fig. 15-18.

Left: Central part. Among the elastin deposits a few tubules but mostly less differentiated "ductal" columns.

Right: Periphery of the tumor with broad cell columns with a tendency to form cribriform structures. The dark cells in the periphery of the cell columns (see Fig. 15-17) are very conspicuous. The cells are otherwise regular and uniform. Mitoses are rather rare. Cell pleomorphism is not typical for tubuloductal carcinomas.

There are also other characteristics. Intraductal growth is usually not prominent in tubuloductal carcinoma, in contrast to comedo cancer.

*Fig. 15-20*

*Tubuloductal carcinoma (tubular carcinoma +) (Invasive ductal carcinoma).* Another example of a tumor classified as tubular carcinoma +. The periphery is very spiculated. Many of the spicules are retracted bands from the surroundings but in some places there is carcinoma growth in the spicules (Bogaert et al., 1977; Linell et al., 1980).

Very prominent eosinophil elastin deposits are seen.

This is a typical example of a stellate cancer. This feature is the hallmark of a tubuloductal tumor, in contrast to the picture of carcinomas of comedo type and other closely related carcinomas (mucinous and medullary carcinoma with lymphoid infiltration), which are polycyclical, circumscribed, "knobby" tumors.

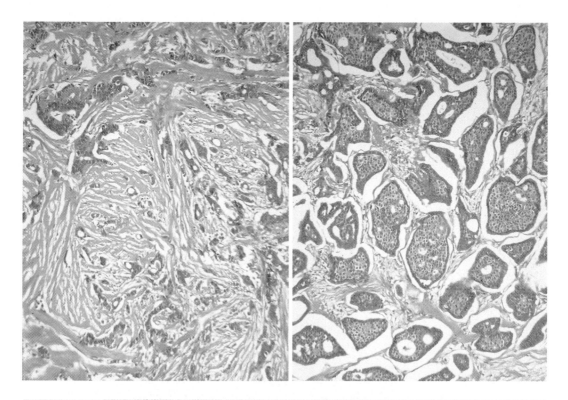

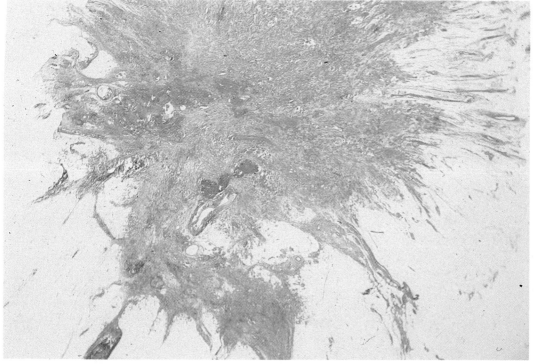

*Fig. 15-21*

*Tubular carcinoma 0 (Invasive ductal carcinoma).* This term denotes that no tubular structures are found, which may certainly be a matter of the extent of the sampling. Otherwise there are no real differences between tubular carcinoma + and 0. The same cell type is seen and there are usually abundant elastin deposits. On the whole we have the same cell type as in other tubuloductal carcinomas. To the left, a central portion of the tumor, showing undifferentiated columns infiltrating the wall of a duct with normal epithelium. This circling of cancerous columns around normal structures is often seen in tubuloductal and lobular carcinomas, but is practically never seen in comedo carcinoma.

To the right, a close-up of the periphery, showing the undifferentiated columns. But the cell type is the same as in the foregoing pictures.

The characteristic spiculated or star-like appearance is more or less lost during tumor progression because of growth of cancer columns between the spicules. This is described in detail by Linell et al. (1980).

*Fig. 15-22*

*Tubuloductal carcinoma (tubular carcinoma +) (Invasive ductal carcinoma).* To the left, part of a carcinoma with abundant elastin deposits in the stroma. Centrally there were a few tubular elements and the carcinoma was classified as tubular carcinoma +. In the lower part there are two spicules containing intraductal tumor growth (arrows). This is sometimes seen, usually at the base of the spicules, which otherwise comprise mostly connective tissue with or without glandular elements, contracted from the surroundings. In between the spicules there is invasive cancer growth out into the fatty tissue (double arrow). Elastin stain.

To the right, a detail of the periphery with columns of cells, rather characteristic of tubuloductal carcinoma. The cells are middle-sized and uniform with rather light cytoplasm. Mitoses are rare.

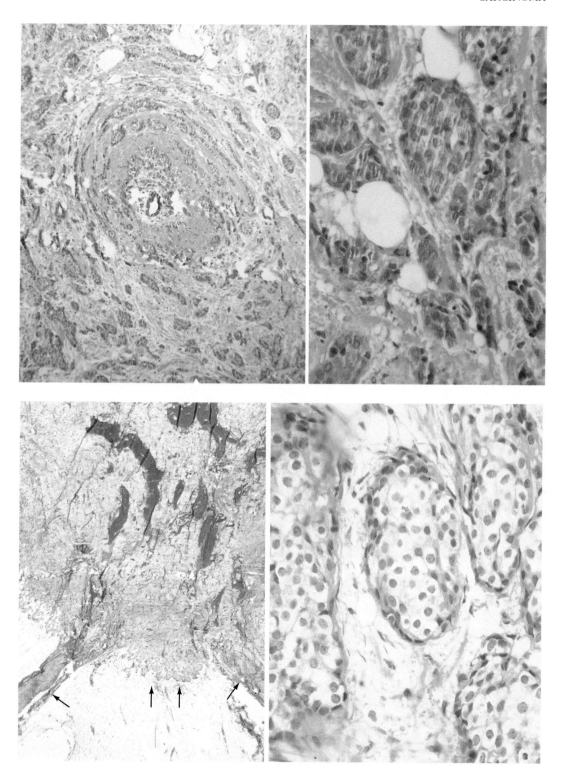

*Fig. 15-23*

*Tubuloductal carcinoma (tubular carcinoma +) (Invasive ductal carcinoma).*

Left: An overview. In the upper part the central area of carcinoma with sclerotic stroma and abundant elastin (eosinophil) especially in duct walls. In the lower part the periphery of the tumor with tumor growth in compact, undifferentiated columns.

Center: The picture is traversed by a broad band of elastin and around it are tubular structures with rather tall epithelium, which may be a sign of tumor progression from the low epithelium in pure tubular carcinoma.

Right: Compact "ductal" carcinoma strands among broad elastin bands. Such a picture can also be found in the centers of tubular carcinoma 0. The only difference between tubular carcinoma + and tubular carcinoma 0 is the absence of tubules in the latter, which may be only a question of sampling. There is probably little real difference. On the other hand, the table (p. 28) with the higher mean diameter speaks for a further progression from tubular carcinoma +.

*Fig. 15-24*

*Progression in tubuloductal carcinoma (Invasive ductal carcinoma).* This is an interesting case that may illustrate the earlier description of progression in tubuloductal carcinoma, that is, a carcinoma of pure tubular type, which, on several places, shows transition to carcinoma of a lesser differentiated "ductal" type.

At lower left, part of the tubular carcinoma with pronounced deposits of elastin. From this carcinoma there is a narrow bridge (arrow) connecting the tubular carcinoma with a small, less differentiated carcinoma. Elastin stain.

To the right, at higher magnification the bridge with tubular carcinoma. In the upper part there is a more undifferentiated part. See Fig. 15-25. Elastin stain.

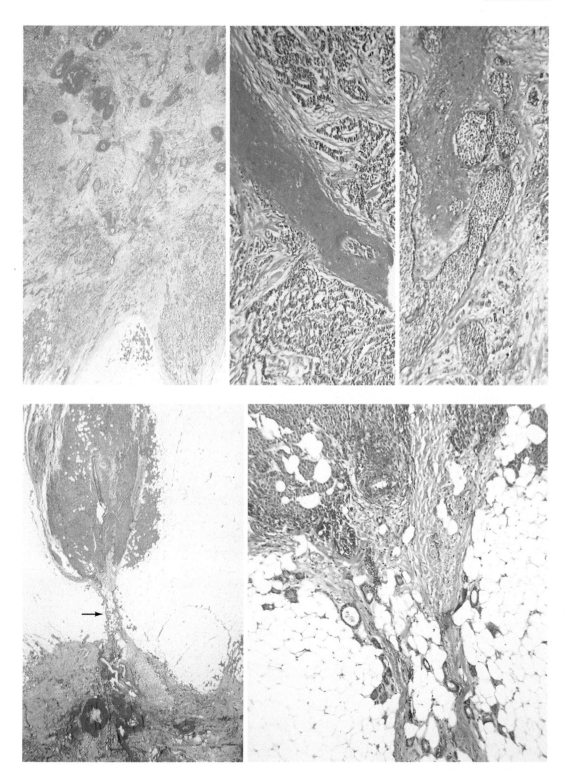

*Fig. 15-25*

*Progression in tubuloductal carcinoma (Invasive ductal carcinoma).* This is a high magnification of parts of Fig. 15-24. To the left, part of the bridge between the parts of the tumor. In this bridge we see a highly differentiated tubular carcinoma. To the right, the less differentiated "ductal" part. Even here, though, the cells are rather monomorphous, growing in solid columns.

See Fig. 15-26.

*Fig. 15-26*

*Progression in tubuloductal carcinoma (Invasive ductal carcinoma).* The explanation given in the text to Figs. 15-24 and 15-25 can be contested. It is conceivable that the close relation between the two types of carcinoma is a consequence of the coalescing of two incidentally adjacent tumors of different types. But this interpretation does not seem very credible on closer study of the tumor. From the central pure tubular carcinoma there are growths of less differentiated carcinoma at several points. In this part such growths of less differentiated tumors are seen in 3-4 separate foci (arrows).

These circumstances seem to support the conception proposed in the text to Fig. 15-24.

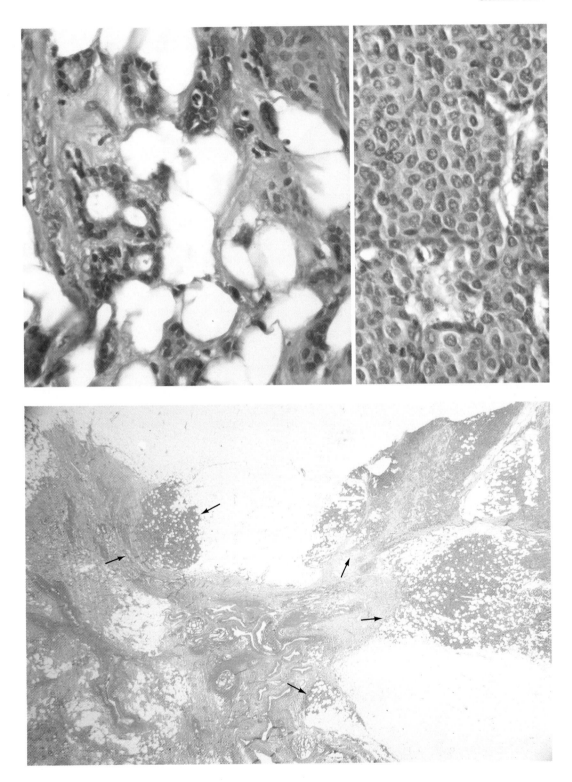

*Fig. 15-27*

*Yellow zone around tubuloductal carcinoma (Invasive ductal carcinoma).* An orange-stained yellow zone is often seen in the border of breast carcinomas. This is characteristic but is practically never seen in any but tubular and tubuloductal carcinomas. We have no proven explanation of this yellow zone. Histologically, usually nothing abnormal is found in the fatty tissue. Sometimes a zone of lipophages can be seen but this is not a constant finding.

The yellow zone is only seen around carcinomas with a strong shrinking tendency and the most probable explanation is that the intense yellow color is caused by a concentration through the shrinking process of yellow-stained substances (lipochromes) in the fatty tissue. This yellow zone, which is best seen in fresh, unfixed specimens, is of very great diagnostic value.

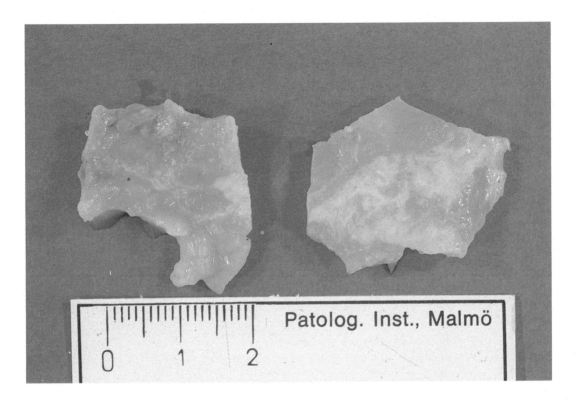

*Fig. 15-28*

*Comedo carcinoma.* Comedo carcinoma has got its name from the dry grayish-yellow cylinders that can be pressed from the cut surface. This can be very clearly seen as grayish-yellow dots in both pictures. It is the gross appearance of the in situ carcinoma that has given the name to this carcinoma. These necrotic cylinders (comedones) may come from solid, cribriform or papillary growths. The term ductal carcinoma of comedo type therefore covers all these types of carcinoma. This is all the more justified as they are often seen in combination, growing side by side. In many classifications papillary carcinoma is treated as a special type. We have never seen a pure papillary carcinoma.

Sooner or later the intraductal carcinoma of comedo type may develop into an infiltrating carcinoma. This may occur in distinct, very small areas, which may be difficult to discern. When infiltration occurs the carcinoma feels much harder. In the following we will illustrate firstly intraductal carcinomas and thereafter cases with infiltrating carcinomas, which generally retain a considerable proportion of intraductal growth.

Macroscopically the comedo carcinomas, besides the comedones, often show a grayish-red, moist cut surface. They are often rather well circumscribed with a polycyclical contour ("knobby" carcinoma).

To the left, a rather well circumscribed tumor with many grayish-white dots. These are the cut ducts filled with carcinoma cells which can be pressed out as "worms". To the right another polycyclically outlined tumor with moist cut surface. In this case the comedones are less conspicuous.

*Fig. 15-29*

*Intraductal comedo carcinoma (Intraductal carcinoma).* This is a very common example of intraductal (in situ carcinoma) of comedo type.

Left: At lower magnification a fatty mammary tissue with fibrous strands containing dilated ducts with carcinoma, growing in micropapillary, cribriform or solid formation on the walls of the ducts, which are surrounded by round cell cuffs. The ducts contain eosinophil masses of debris and necrotic cancer cells.

The necrotic cancer masses often show calcifications and branched calcifications are one of the most significant mammographic findings in comedo cancer. In this case there were no calcifications and no mammographic changes. Fine needle aspiration showed carcinoma and at operation there was very widespread intraductal carcinoma. Why necroses in some carcinomas calcify and others do not, we do not know.

Right: Another part of the same tumor. A duct is filled with compact cancer masses. In the lower part there is a lobule where the end tubules are filled with atypical cells. This is called cancerization of lobules or cancerous outgrowth into lobules. It has even been named "secondary lobular carcinoma in situ". Earlier, such lesions were often interpreted as infiltrating growth.

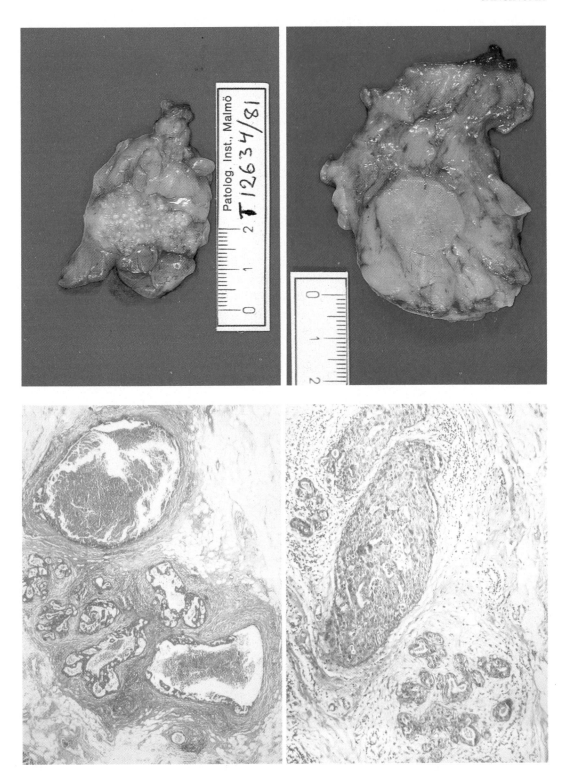

*Fig. 15-30*

*Intraductal carcinoma with different patterns side by side.* Left: Intraductal carcinoma with papillary pattern of different types. In some places there are fibrous stalks in the papillomas. It is sometimes urged that a fibrous core in papillomas denotes a benign lesion, but this does not hold true in all cases. In the lower part (arrows) there are "Roman bridges", structures that Azzopardi feels are highly typical of intraductal carcinoma. In the middle, Roman bridges, combined with papillary and ring-like structures.

Right: High magnification of epithelium seen in the middle (arrow). There is irregular piling up of cells and a moderate atypia.

*Fig. 15-31*

*Intraductal carcinoma of predominantly papillary type.* In the lumen of the ducts necrotic masses (comedo cancer). To the left, in the fatty tissue there are fibrous strands with dilated ducts containing typical intraductal carcinoma. Such changes are often difficult to discern for the naked eye.

To the right, higher magnification of the duct walls with papillary projections resembling bunches of grapes. In this case there were numerous calcifications.

On purely descriptive grounds we call a case as this one "papillary intraductal cancer" but we would like to add: "of comedo type", to stress its status as a subgroup of the comedo carcinomas.

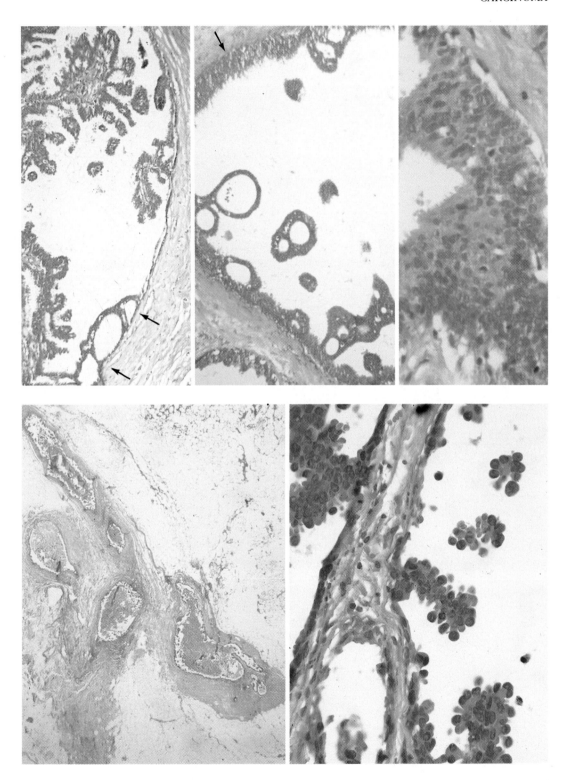

Fig. 15-32

*Intraductal carcinoma (mural or clinging type).* This is from a 40-year-old woman who complained of a lump in the lower part of her breast. A biopsy showed only fatty tissue on gross examination. A very experienced pathologist did not notice anything exceptional when he cut throught the fatty tissue, which had been crumpled up in too small a jar. All tissue was embedded and histologic examination revealed several small islands of the type shown to the left lying in the fatty tissue. This is a tiny piece of connective tissue containing a cluster of widened ducts lined by basophil epithelium with micropapillary structures.

To the right, a detail (arrow in the picture on the left) showing the atypical multi-layered epithelium where many cells have "apocrine snouts". A curious papilla with a ring structure is seen at the top.

Fig. 15-33

*Intraductal carcinoma of mural or "clinging" type.* "Clinging" is difficult to translate into other languages. It can be described as climbing on a wall, as ivy does. "Mural" (also proposed by Azzopardi) seems to be a more current term internationally.

To the left, a cluster of dilated ducts with thick hyalinized walls. Macroscopically the specimen looked like macaroni. Large parts of the walls are devoid of epithelium, but scattered, irregular epithelium (arrows) lines the ducts.

To the right, a close-up of one of the arrowed details with a "Roman bridge" and a papillary outgrowth of highly atypical epithelium.

We do not know if this case represents an incipient intraductal carcinoma or a remnant after desquamation and attempt at self-healing of an intraductal carcinoma (cf. Ch. 15).

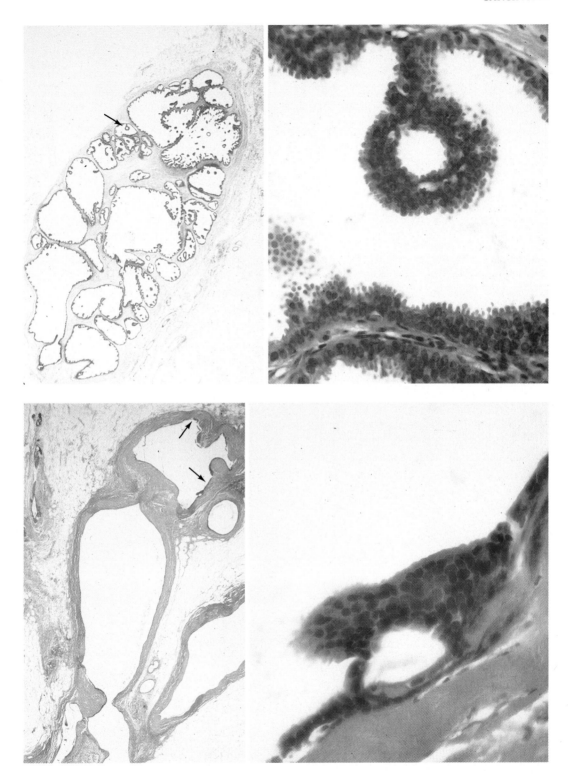

*Fig. 15-34*

*Mural intraductal carcinoma with preserved myothelium.* The picture to the left shows dilated ducts with a micropapillary mural carcinoma. Some of the papillae are very long and slender and often cut obliquely, therefore sometimes appearing as separate islands. Already at this magnification a basal myothelial cell layer can be discerned.

The picture to the right shows a detail of the atypical multi-layered epithelium exhibiting micropapillary structures. But the preserved myothelial layer is also clearly seen. The picture is intended to show that the dogmatic view, i.e. that the preserved myothelial layer is a proof of a benign lesion, is not valid in all situations.

*Fig. 15-35*

*Ductal carcinoma of comedo type (Invasive ductal carcinoma).* This case illustrates difficulties which may occur in interpreting the pictures of carcinomas of comedo type. At bottom right, a lobule with cancerization. This is *not* infiltration. To the right there is clear infiltrative growth into the fatty tissue. To the left, an area where probably most of the growth represents cancerization of lobules with round cell infiltration in the stroma. It may be extremely difficult to decide whether there is a true infiltration in this area. This problem is also encountered on an ultrastructural level (Ozello, 1971)

At lower left there is a cancer column (arrow), which may represent growth in a lymph vessel, although the space seen around the cluster of cancer cells may also be an artifact.

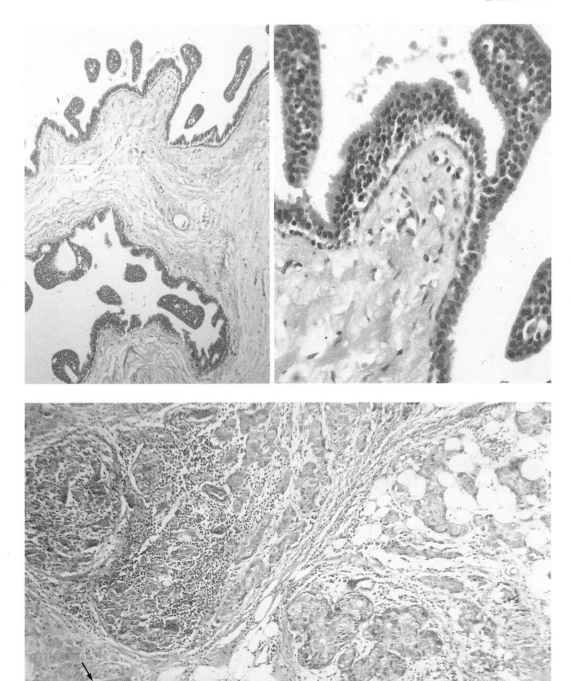

*Fig. 15-36*

*Intraductal carcinoma.* This is another example of earlier misinterpretation. The patient was a 22-year-old nurse with lumpiness in the left breast and yellow secretion. During a period of 2 years four local excisions were performed and interpreted as benign "fibroadenosis". The picture is illustrated here.

Left: At the upper right, intraductal carcinoma. In the lower part of the picture there are normal lobules and cancerization of lobules. Right: Detail of the picture on the left.

The slides were revised as intraductal carcinoma. A bilateral subcutaneous mastectomy was done. The right breast was normal but the left revealed widespread intraductal carcinoma and in a few, very small, places there was beginning infiltration. The patient is still well after 10 years.

*Fig. 15-37*

*Intraductal carcinoma with multiple infiltration.* Intraductal carcinomas may be widespread in the breast. They may occupy large parts of the breast or appear as multiple foci which may be more or less scattered. Intraductal carcinomas may be extremely widespread and still show no signs of infiltration.

Infiltrative growth often occurs as multiple, mostly small, foci. It may be very difficult to find these foci and an extensive and adequate sampling is always to be recommended in intraductal carcinoma. Sometimes areas of infiltration are found macroscopically as multiple hard foci.

Left: Part of intraductal carcinoma with cribriform and papillary structures.

Center: At the top a part of a duct with bridging and papillary carcinoma. At the bottom, infiltrating carcinoma growing in solid columns.

Right: Part of intraductal growth. The carcinoma shows atypical cells but the cellular polymorphism is not especially pronounced.

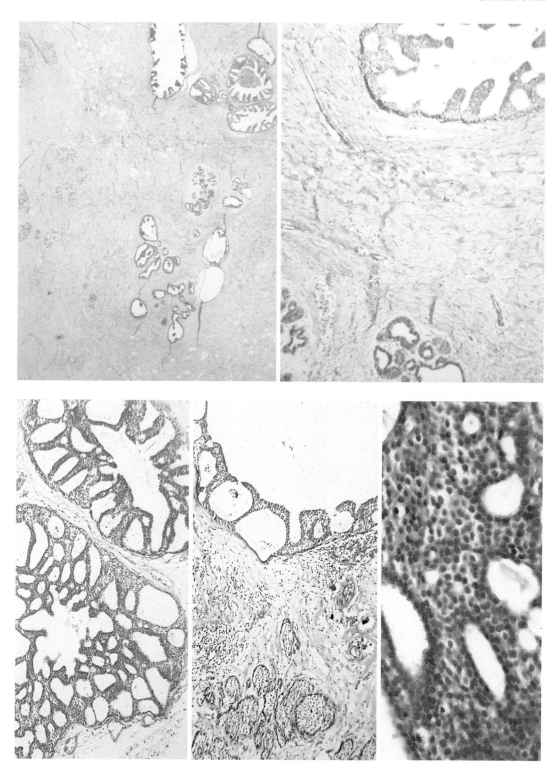

*Fig. 15-38*

*Ductal carcinoma of comedo type with glandular infiltration (Invasive ductal carcinoma).* This is a very interesting and rather rare type of comedo carcinoma. The intraductal part is mostly cribriform but made up of large polymorphous cells. The infiltrative component shows the picture of adenocarcinoma. The glandular structures are lined by large, cylindric cells with pronounced atypia. This type of comedo carcinoma should not be confused with tubular carcinoma (Linell et al., 1980). See next picture.

This type of comedo carcinoma is also particularly mentioned in the last edition of WHO nomenclature.

Left: Mostly intraductal growth of cribriform carcinoma, comprising large polymorphous cells.

Right: In the upper right hand corner a dilated duct with cribriform cancer with large central necrosis. The rest of the picture is occupied by infiltrating cancer growing as an adenocarcinoma with glandlike structures lined with tall atypical epithelium.

*Fig. 15-39*

*Ductal carcinoma of comedo type with glandular infiltration (Invasive ductal carcinoma).* Left: Part of intraductal carcinoma with (in the upper part) a classic picture of comedo carcinoma: a solid proliferation with a large central necrosis. In the lower part, another duct with a more papillary-cribriform pattern of the cancerous growth.

Center: The infiltrative carcinoma with irregular adenocarcinomatous structures. Right: At higher magnification, showing the highly polymorphous epithelium. Several mitoses are seen.

This case illustrates how closely related different types of intraductal carcinomas are. Besides the cribriform pattern the intraductal component also contains solid carcinoma and the infiltrative component forms glandlike structures.

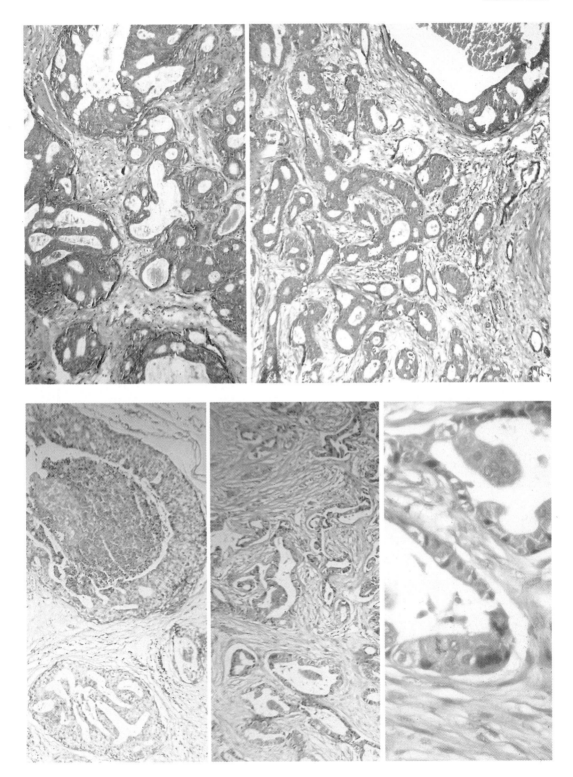

*Fig. 15-40*

*Ductal carcinoma of apocrine type.* In our opinion this is a variant of comedo carcinoma with cells exhibiting features of apocrini. There is abundant eosinophil granular cytoplasm of the same type seen in apocrine metaplasia in cystic breast lesions (see Fig. 14-1).

To the left, clustered ducts lined by this type of epithelium. The lumina are filled with debris from desquamated necrotic cells.

To the right, a detail showing the large granular eosinophil cells with nuclei having large nucleoli. The atypia is moderate.

Most authorities (Hamperl, 1977) agree that ductal carcinoma with apocrine traits (total or partial) does not differ in its behavior from other types of comedo carcinomas.

*Fig. 15-41*

*Infiltrating ductal carcinoma of comedo type with mucin production.* This is to exemplify another sub-type of comedo carcinoma with special traits, i.e. mucin production. As we have mentioned earlier, comedo carcinomas and "mucinous carcinomas" may have many features in common. Tumors which are only partially mucin producing usually show in other parts the same structure as common comedo carcinomas. To the left, an area consistent with comedo carcinoma with intraductal component in the upper field: around this duct there is infiltration of solid carcinoma columns. To the right, mucinous formation with carcinoma columns floating in mucin; that is, the same picture that is found overall in a pure mucinous carcinoma.

Varying degrees of mucin production may occur in all kinds of breast carcinoma (see under Mucinous carcinoma, Ch. 15).

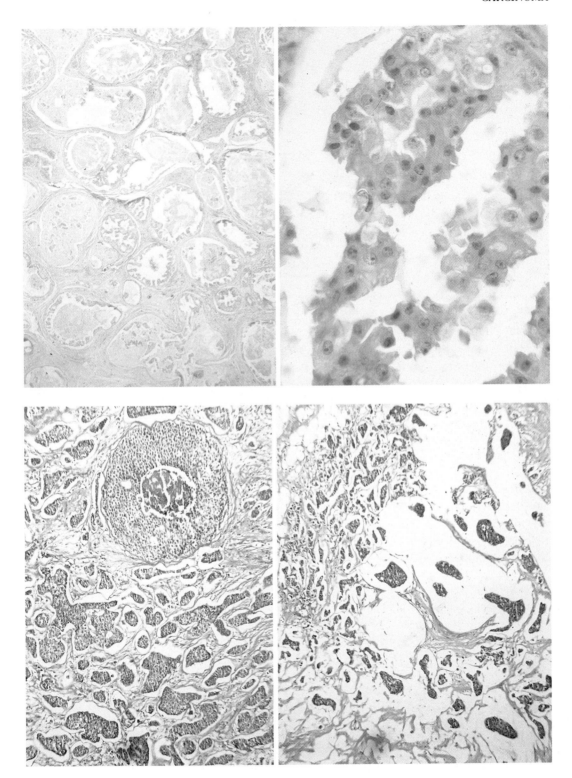

*Fig. 15-42*

*Intraductal carcinoma with intralymphatic spread.* This is a very rare finding. To the left there is an intraductal carcinoma with a cribriform and papillary pattern.

To the right the same type of carcinoma is growing in lymphatic vessels. In this case a very extensive search for invasive carcinoma was instituted, with negative results. Naturally there may have been small foci of invasive growth which were not found, and which could be the explanation. Normally we do not accept the idea of intralymphatic growth in an intraductal carcinoma. But we should also realize the possibility that there is no sharp distinction between in situ growth and invasion (ultrastructure research by Ozello, 1971). Such studies have revealed that the border between the intraductal growth and the surrounding tissue is not as sharp as is often believed and that the basal membrane may rupture. Such phenomena may explain some of the cases with axillary metastases without apparent invasive component in the breast (Rosen, 1980).

*Fig. 15-43*

*Where do comedo carcinomas (Ductal carcinoma) start?* In his brilliant studies on the origins of breast carcinomas Muir came to the conclusion that ductal carcinoma (the type we call comedo cancer) begins as atypical cell proliferations intraductally. His description still seems valid with the exception that nowadays we describe ducts and tubules somewhat different than Muir. There is no doubt that we find the earliest stages of comedo carcinoma as intraductal proliferations in groups of ducts and probably as a progression from epitheliosis. These groups of ducts Wellings et al., 1975 explain as "outfolding" of lobules in terminal ductolobular units. The end tubules of the lobules are dilated and reduced in number. This conception was developed by Wellings & Jensen in comprehensive studies and it is highly probable that it gives a truer picure of the events. The groups of cysts in mastopathia cystica are essentially the same as "AL" (atypical lobule) with more or less atypical epithelial proliferation.

To the left, a group of "ducts" filled with epithelial proliferations. But only two of the ducts have elastin in the walls. The other "ducts" have no elastin and are probably derived from lobular tubules, dilated in outfolding of the terminal ductolobular unit.

To the right, a detail showing a duct with elastin in the wall. Both the duct and the adjacent duct derived from a lobule are filled with moderately atypical epithelial cells. Transformation to foam cells is also seen (arrow).

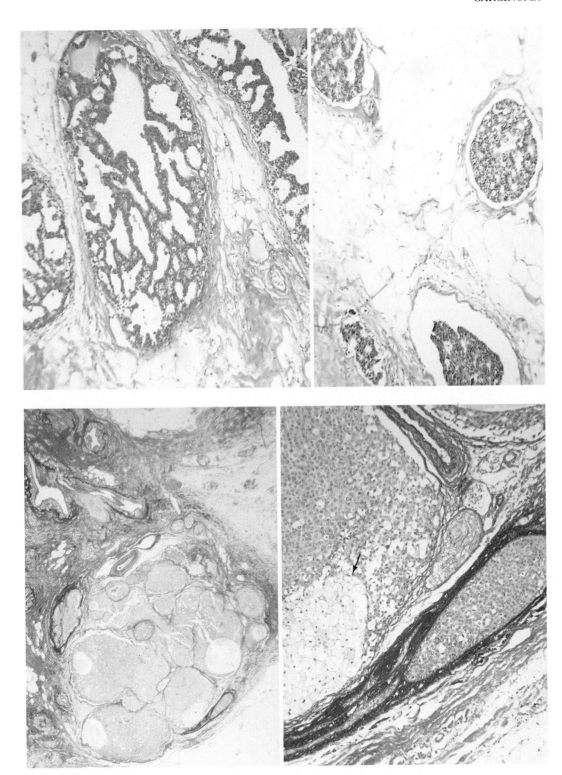

*Fig.15-44*

*Intracystic carcinoma.* Left: Part of a cystic lesion filled with papillary masses with moderately atypical epithelial cells on slender fibrous stalks.

Right: Detail of the lower part with suspicion of invasion of the capsule.

This case from a 61-year-old woman was initially diagnosed as a benign papilloma. Four years later the patient presented with a 3×2-cm-large tumor in the same place. It was a hemorrhagic papillomatous tumor with the same pattern but with clearcut invasion.

This is an example of highly differentiated papillary intracystic carcinoma, often diagnosed as benign papilloma. Tumors of this type are to be looked upon as carcinoma in situ. They rarely metastasize or recur locally. They are often seen in rather old women and the prognosis is mostly excellent. Therefore it often does not matter if they are called benign. Wide local excision seems to be an adequate therapy.

*Fig.15-45*

*Intracystic carcinoma.* This is another example of a tumor much like that in Fig.15-44.

Left: Hemorrhagic tumor with very slender papillae with tall, moderately atypical cylindric cells.

Right: Detail of the bottom part. There is suspicion of invasion into the capsule.

This case is rather similar to the one in the foregoing picture. Intracystic carcinoma is mammographically a well circumscribed lesion much like a cyst, although it cannot be emptied by puncture. It can readily be diagnosed cytologically, but if it is very highly differentiated, the cytologic diagnosis is difficult as is also the histologic diagnosis. It must be admitted that there is no sharp distinction between papillomas and intracystic carcinomas.

We look upon intracystic carcinoma as a variant of comedo carcinoma. This view is also justified by the fact that intracystic carcinoma may show the same variations (solid, cribriform growth, etc.) as other comedo carcinomas. On the other hand, intracystic carcinoma has a much better prognosis than common comedo carcinomas, probably because it remains at an in situ stage for a long time.

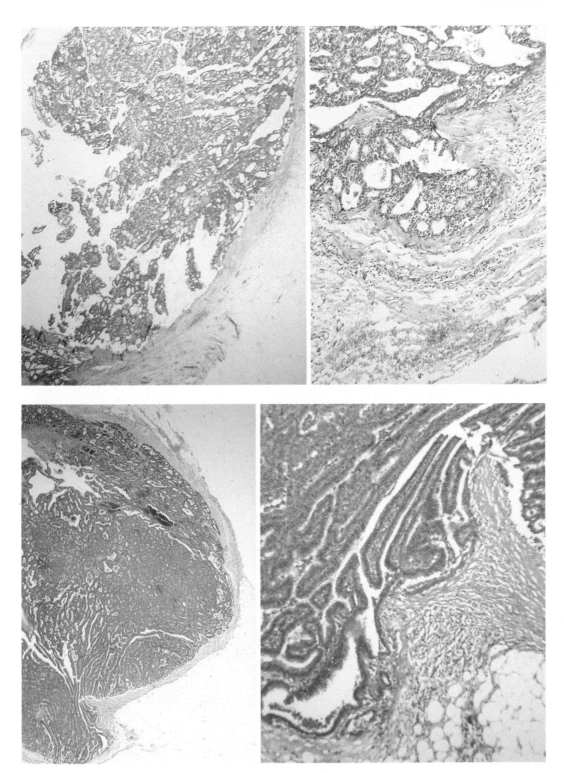

*Fig. 15-46*

*Mucinous (colloid) carcinoma*. The specimen is from a 62-year-old woman. The picture shows a polycyclic, rather well delineated (knobby) tumor with a glistening cut surface. At incision one often gets mucinous material on the knife, which is highly characteristic.

Around the tumor there are adipose tissue and breast parenchyma, rather abundant considering to the age of the patient.

To the right another case with islands of adipose tissue intermingled with the glistening tumor-growth.

*Fig. 15-47*

*Mucinous (colloid) carcinoma*. This is a rather typical case of pure mucinous carcinoma. The pure mucinous carcinoma is characterized by large mucinous lakes of mostly acid mucins. In these lakes there are floating epithelial aggregates, which may show compact or glandular structures. This type of mucinous carcinoma is said to be common in old women. It carries a relatively good prognosis. Most carcinomas in old women tend to have a good prognosis because the patient tends to die from other causes before the cancer has had time to kill.

It is said that the good prognosis is correlated with the mucinous character. Only cancers which are exclusively mucinous in type show this favorable prognosis. This is certainly a question of sampling. When you cut several blocks from a mucinous carcinoma you will find parts without mucin production and these parts look like common carcinoma of comedo type. Intraductal carcinoma in the vicinity mostly shows comedo type.

Therefore we are of the opinion that mucinous carcinoma is a variant of ductal carcinoma of comedo type and should be regarded as a subgroup thereof.

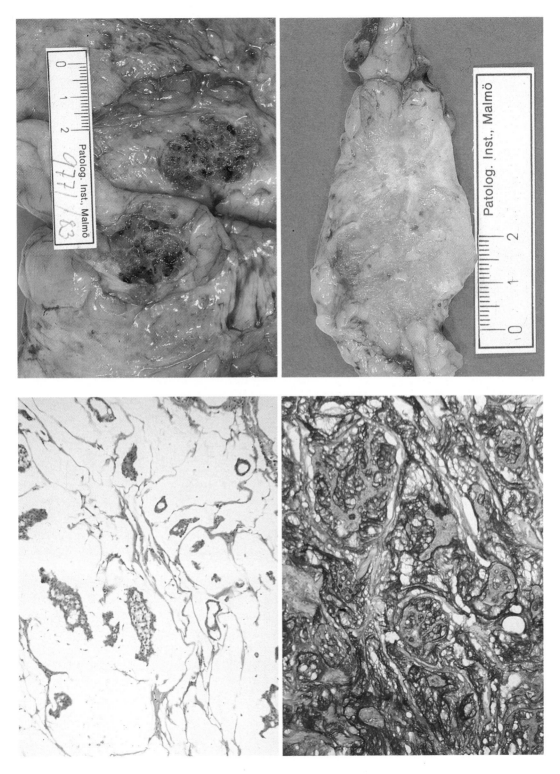

*Fig. 15-48*

*Mucinous (colloid) carcinoma*. These are details from the foregoing case.

To the left, aggregates of cancer cells floating in mucin, not stained by hematoxylin-eosin. The cells are rather polymorphous. They are surrounded by mucin but also contain intracytoplasmatic mucin (light cytoplasm).

To the right, in the upper field, abundant mucin. In the lower field, little mucin production; the cancer looks exactly like an infiltrating (ductal) carcinoma of comedo type. Alcian-blue-PAS staining.

With adequate and plentiful sampling we do not think that any truly pure mucinous carcinomas would be found.

*Fig. 15-49*

*Mucin production of tubuloductal carcinoma (Mucin production of invasive ductal carcinoma)*. All kinds of breast carcinomas can produce mucin. As we have already pointed out, the mucinous carcinoma should probably be looked upon as a variant of carcinoma of comedo type. But sometimes abundant mucin production is also encountered in typical tubuloductal carcinomas, although rarely.

To the left, a typical tubuloductal carcinoma of what we call tubular carcinoma + + (see Ch. 15). Tubular structures are seen to be combined with less differentiated "ductal" structures. At the lower left there is abundant mucin production (arrow) with aggregates of cancer cells floating in mucin (not stained).

To the right a detail stained in Alcian-blue-PAS showing groups of cancer cells floating in the acid mucin masses.

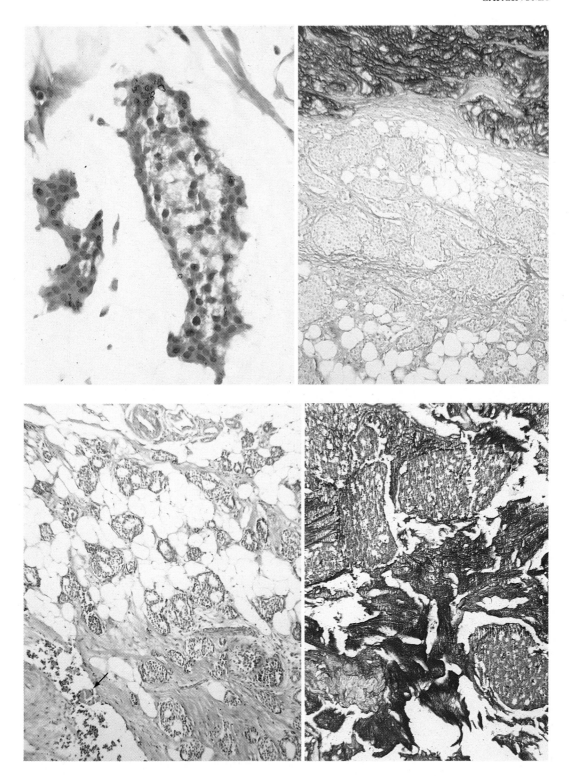

*Fig. 15-50*

*Signet ring cell carcinoma*. This is another type of mucin producing carcinoma. We will illustrate and discuss this type later in Ch. 15 but wish to remind the reader of this rare type of carcinoma, which is said to have a sinister prognosis.

To the left, a view of the cancer with the cells arranged in alveolar structures. The cells have excentric nuclei and light eosinophil cytoplasm, sometimes with vacuoles.

To the right, in Alcian-blue-PAS staining, numerous mucin drops in the cells.

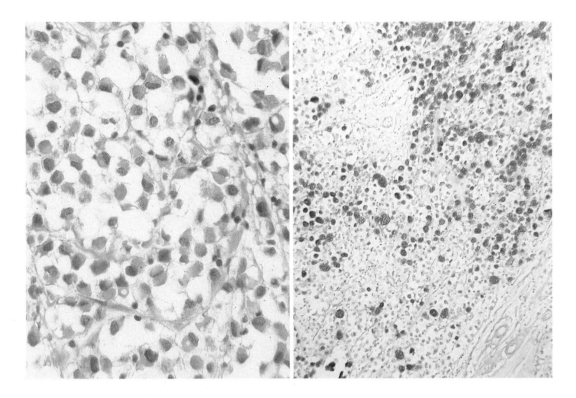

*Fig. 15-51*

*Medullary carcinoma with lymphoid stroma infiltration.* This tumor has been distinguished as a special type. The name "medullary" was much in use formerly and is still used for more than it deserves. Many "medullary" carcinomas are only partly medullary, often having sclerotic central parts. The type described here is mostly medullary throughout. The typical case with lymphoid infiltration is a well delineated, rather soft tumor with a reddish-gray cut surface which often shows more or less prominent yellow necroses.

In our opinion tumors of this category are closely related to comedo carcinoma, forming a spectrum of types according to the degree of lymphoid infiltration. Classic medullary carcinoma with abundant lymphoid infiltration may thus be regarded as one extreme of this spectrum and medullary carcinoma devoid of such an infiltration (i.e. comedo carcinoma) as the other extreme.

The picture shows a rather well circumscribed tumor with yellow necroses.

*Fig. 15-52*

*Medullary carcinoma with lymphoid stroma infiltration.* This is a typical case. Left: The border of the tumor. We see a fibrous capsule in the upper part of the picture (arrows). Such fibroblastic proliferation at the border of the tumor is often seen and justifies the name "circumscribed carcinoma" (Haagensen). In the lower part of the picture, part of the tumor with columns of large cells intermingled with strands of lymphocytes and plasma cells. Center: A close-up of the large polymorphous cells intimately connected to the inflammatory infiltrate, which often consists of more plasma cells than lymphocytes.

Right: Alcian-blue-PAS stained tumor tissue showing mucous substances (blue) between the cells and also target shaped mucinous "drops" in the cells. Such mucinous deposits may be absent.

This case is an example of classic medullary carcinoma but when the lympho-plasmo-cellular infiltration is more scanty or patchy the structure of the tumor may generally conform with a common comedo carcinoma.

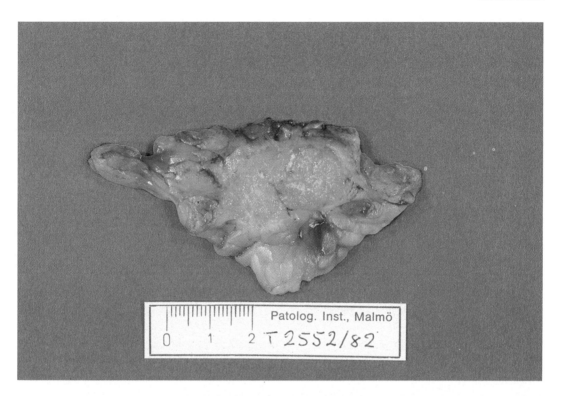

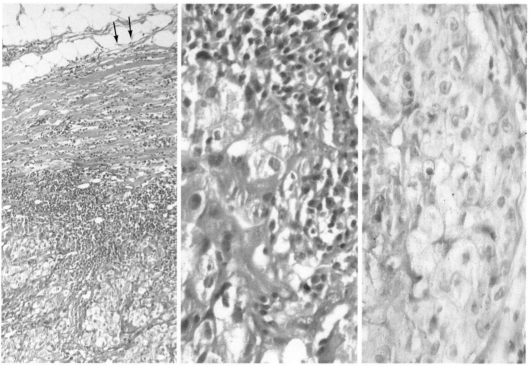

*Fig. 15-53*

*Medullary carcinoma with lymphoid stroma infiltration.* This is another case of the same type. Left: The sharp delimitation of the tumor can be seen, although there is an outer zone of round cell infiltration among narrow infiltrating strands of tumor (arrows).

Right: On the left hand side, a large eosinophil coagulation necrosis. On the right, a vital part of the tumor with medullary columns separated by narrow strands of round cells. The tumor here is well circumscribed.

These tumors have much in common with the comedo carcinomas. The large polymorphous cells are common for both. An intraductal comedo component may occur in medullary carcinoma with lymphoid stroma infiltration.

*Fig. 15-54*

*Medullary carcinoma with lymphoid stroma infiltration. Lymph node metastases.* This is from the same case as in the foregoing picture. Left: A picture of a lymph node, practically filled with a metastasis, which shows widespread spontaneous necrosis in the center. Right: A close-up of the necrosis, consisting of shadows of tumor cells. The necrosis is surrounded by foreign body giant cells and, more peripherally, fibroblasts and histiocytes. This feature is a characteristic of medullary carcinoma. It may be speculated that this reaction is the result of immunologic processes.

It has been argued (Bloom et al., 1970) that medullary carcinoma with lymphoid infiltration has a much better prognosis than other carcinomas; others do not share this opinion. The differences may be due to difficulties in classification.

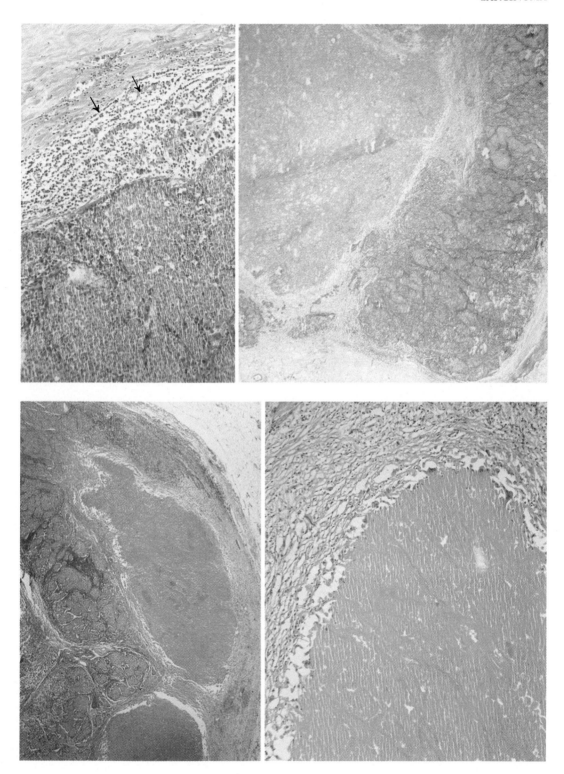

*Fig. 15-55*

*Lobular carcinoma in situ.* What we call infiltrating lobular carcinoma today has been known for a long time under various designations (small cell carcinoma, scirrhous carcinoma). Lobular carcinoma in situ (Lcis or Clis = Carcinoma lobulare in situ) had already been described in the 1890's.

In the twenties Ewing described it as a precancerous stage, but it was the work of Foote & Stewart in the forties that made this condition general knowledge. It took, however, a very long time, almost until the seventies, for this lesion to be accepted as a cancerous or precancerous lesion and there is still much debate about the exact nature of this lesion.

Lobular carcinoma in situ (Lcis) has a highly characteristic appearance. The end tubules in one or more lobules are expanded by compact rounded aggregates of uniform, rather small cells.

To the left, an agglomeration of lobules with changes. In the larger ducts there are often changes of the same type. In a cross-section they resemble a bunch of grapes but in long section they look like a duct filled with cells (in the middle).

To the right, a higher magnification with the end tubules filled with small monomorphous cells with rather small nuclei and small distinct nucleoli. Mitoses are very rarely seen.

*Fig. 15-56*

*Lobular carcinoma in situ.* Branching ducts with Lcis can show a complicated, tree-like, highly characteristic pattern. For these duct changes the name pagetoid changes has been used, but this term should be abandoned because the cells in Lcis mainly grow in continuous aggregations and "pagetoid" spread is a less conspicuous feature.

In the picture we see branching ducts with a pronounced proliferation of small regular cells in several layers. The lumen lining epithelium is atrophic or desquamated. The groups of proliferating cells often look like bunches of grapes (arrows). The picture is highly characteristic.

200

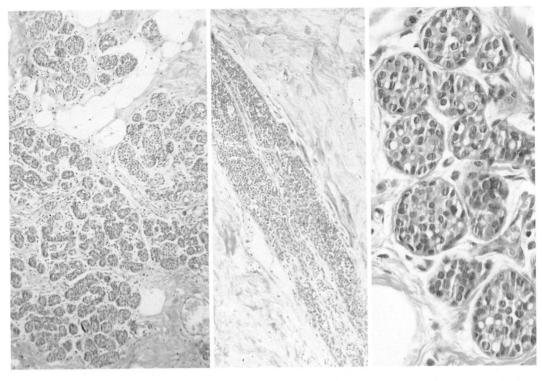

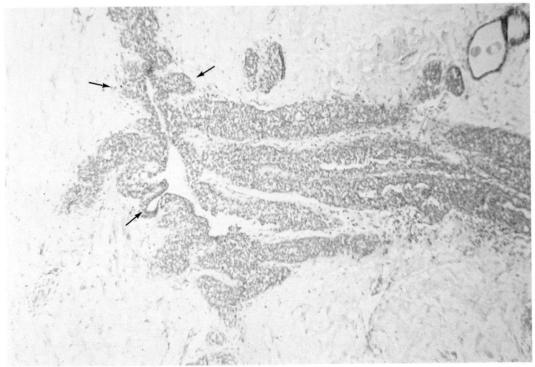

*Fig. 15-57*

*Lobular carcinoma in situ.* To the left, a duct with basal proliferations of uniform cells of the type seen in Lcis. The cells grow as rounded, well demarcated agglomerations. The cells have small vesicular nuclei with delicate nucleoli. Towards the lumen there is a layer of very shallow atrophic epithelium cells which probably represents the original normal epithelium (arrows). To the right, a lobule with the end tubules expanded by monomorphic regular cells. At one place (arrow) there is a remnant of the normal epithelium. See the next figure. The cells are very regular, with monomorphous small nuclei. Different types of Lcis have been described (Haagensen): Type A with small nuclei and type B with larger and more polymorphous nuclei. Haagensen et al. dislike the name lobular carcinoma in situ, preferring the term lobular neoplasia.

*Fig. 15-58*

*Lobular carcinoma in situ.* In this case the original, normal epithelium partly persists in lobules involved by Lcis. The dominating cells from Lcis grow outside the normal epithelium and it is tempting to assume that the cells in Lcis are derived from myothelium (Hamperl). This idea has been defeated by results from histochemical studies showing actin in a cell-layer outside the neoplastic cells in Lcis. It has been argued that it is therefore impossible for the neoplastic cells to be derived from the myothelial cells. This may not, however, constitute real proof because it is possible that neoplastic myothelial cells may have lost their actin. The question of the histogenesis of Lcis must await further investigation.

To the left, a ductolobular unit with light neoplastic cells and small remnants of the normal epithelium (arrows). This is more conspicuous to the right at higher magnification, where arrows point to the epithelium remnants.

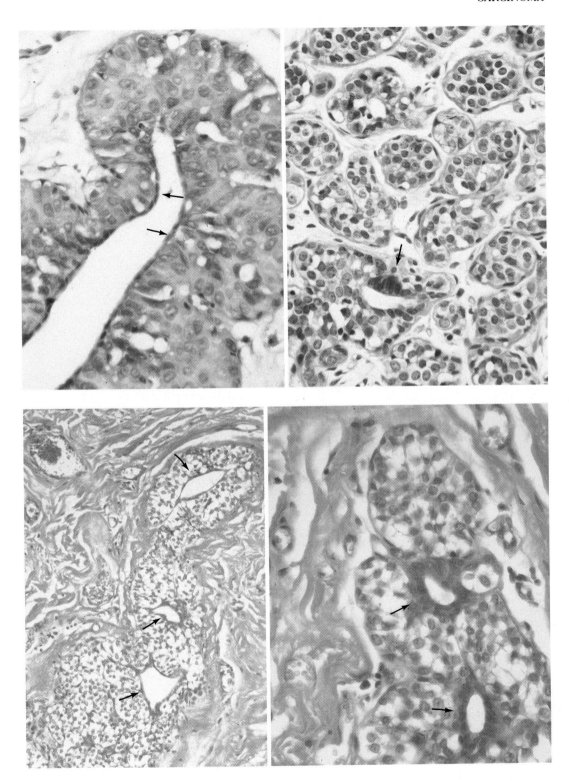

*Fig. 15-59*

*Infiltrating lobular carcinoma.* This tumor type is believed to represent the invasive form of lobular carcinoma. The infiltration is usually diffuse and the tumor cells generally grow in narrow rows ("Indian files"). These often encircle preserved ducts.

The cells are small and often show targetoid mucin drops, which are believed to be infoldings of glycocalyx (Eusebi et al., 1977). This latter feature is not pathognomonic but can be seen in varying degrees in all kinds of breast carcinomas.

Left: Lcis near an infiltrating lobular carcinoma, seen in the middle. The narrow rows of tumor cells encircle a normal duct with preserved, normal two-layer epithelium. Right: An area of the tumor, stained with Alcian-blue-PAS at high magnification, showing mucin drops, often targetoid.

This is the common type of what we call infiltrating lobular carcinoma. In a high percentage of cases foci of lobular carcinoma in situ are found in close proximity to the infiltrating tumor. We have never seen a direct continuity between cancer in situ and infiltrating carcinoma. It is interesting that infiltrating lobular carcinoma very often shows abundant elastin deposits, which are never found in relation to lobular carinoma in situ. This is one of many enigmas in lobular carcinoma.

*Fig. 15-60*

*Metastases of lobular carcinoma.* The metastases of lobular carcinoma have a highly characteristic picture, the cells growing diffusely in a manner reminiscent of a malignant lymphoma.

To the left, part of a lymph node with central lipomatosis. The parenchyma is almost completely replaced by tumor cells. To the right the cells show diffuse infiltration. The cells are small and monomorphous, just as in the primary tumor. This type of metastatic growth is characteristic for lobular carcinoma and very helpful in diagnosis of cases where the classification of the primary tumor is uncertain.

Sometimes the metastases of lobular carcinoma show up in another way (see Fig. 15-96).

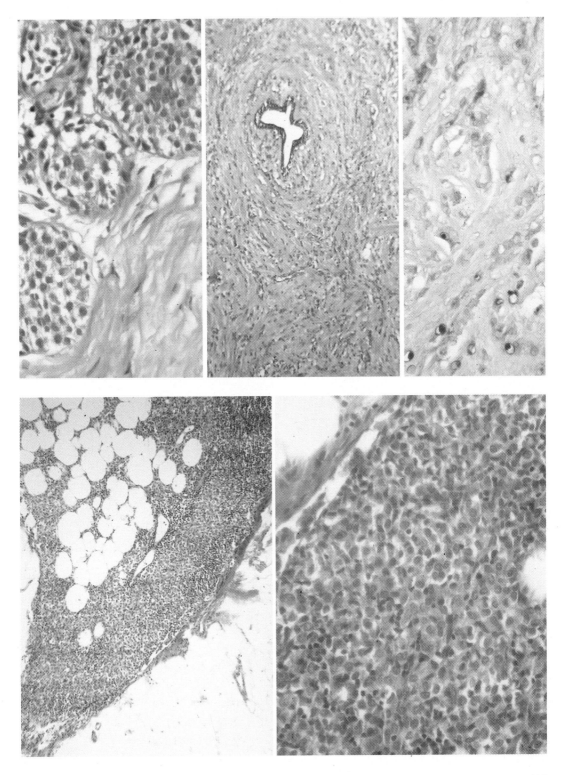

*Fig. 15-61*

*Lobular carcinoma in situ (atrophic or meager type).* Lcis is often described as an expansion of the end tubules or ducts, which look larger than in normal lobules. This is not always seen. Sometimes the end tubules are very narrow, although filled with small monomorphous cells.

The three pictures here show an example of such a case. At the higher magnification on the right the cells are loosely arranged, probably because it is a necropsy specimen with some autolysis.

This is a type of lobular carcinoma in situ which many pathologists have had difficulties accepting. However, this may occur in connection with infiltrating lobular carcinoma and there are no indications that this type would be an innocent lesion.

*Fig. 15-62*

*Delusive lobular carcinoma in situ.* Atrophic or meager Lcis may cause diagnostic difficulties. This picture shows an example. To the left, a structure which may show a superficial resemblance to structures in Fig. 15-61.

At a higher magnification (to the right) one can see that the seemingly haphazardly arranged cells can form glandlike or tubular structures and obviously constitute normal lobules and ducts with light atrophic epithelium (arrows).

The type of atrophic Lcis in ducts and lobules is often seen in old women. Atrophic lobular carcinoma in situ is also mostly seen in older patients. It is possible that both the real and the delusive lobular carcinoma in situ are exponents for the same type of atrophic changes in old women.

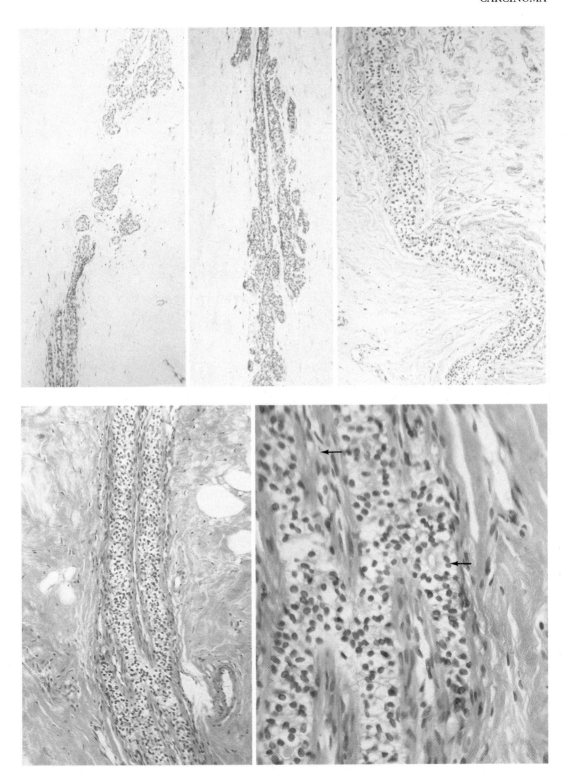

*Fig. 15-63*

*Infiltrating lobular carcinoma.* The atrophic type of Lcis is not accepted as a carcinoma by all pathologists, probably because it looks rather innocent. The specimen shown in this picture comes from a case of subcutaneous mastectomy. The entire specimen was sliced, embedded and sectioned. It contained many foci of Lcis of the atrophic type, but only in two very small foci, which are wholly contained in the pictures, there was infiltrating carcinoma. In the picture to the right is a structure of Lcis of atrophic type (arrow).

*Fig. 15-64*

*Early lobular carcinoma in situ.* Lobular carcinoma in situ is evidently made up of cells from outside the lumen-lining epithelium. In the early stages remnants of this epithelium persist (see Fig. 15-58). During this time it can be mistaken for "lobular atypia". In such cases it is helpful to find typical full-grown lobules with Lcis. Such is the case in this example. Left: On the right one can see parts of normal lobules but on the left two lobules show proliferation of cells beneath the lining epithelium. If transitional forms between this type and unequivocal Lcis are identified, the diagnosis is easy.

If we do not see any clearcut pictures of Lcis the differential diagnosis from lobular atypia may be difficult. In the latter condition however, we have epithelial proliferation with tall epithelial cells (Ch. 14). It is important to note that we often meet this type of lobular atypia in close connection with Lcis.

It has frequently been stated that the diagnosis Lcis should not be made unless there are at least three lobules with typical changes. Naturally this is illogical and unacceptable. The diagnosis is founded on histologic changes independent of the amount of changes.

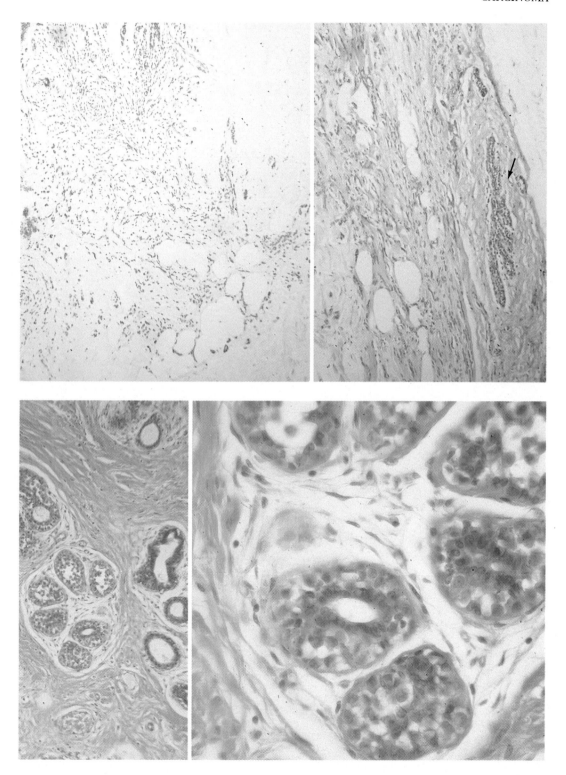

*Fig. 15-65*

*Infiltrating lobular carcinoma.* The finding of Lcis in close connection to infiltrating lobular carcinoma is considered to be the reason for classifying them together but we seldom or never see an outburst of the cells in Lcis forming the infiltrating type. Left: A couple of lobules with typical Lcis. In the surrounding stroma we see the infiltrating strands. Center: Infiltrating strand encircling a normal duct. Right: carcinoma cells with mucin drops.

The difficulty in finding a direct transition between Lcis and the infiltrating carcinoma is one of the reasons why Lcis is such a vexing question. Foote & Stewart argued for an aggressive attitude towards Lcis, which has been followed by a more conservative attitude. There seems to be general agreement that the finding of Lcis implies a substantially increased risk of getting an infiltrating carcinoma. Figures as high as a 10 fold risk have appeared but these are disputed. Moreover, the infiltrating carcinoma occurs with the same frequency on the ipsilateral as on the contralateral side. And only half of the carcinomas are lobular. This has led to the idea that Lcis is not a real carcinoma in situ but rather a marker for forthcoming malignancy. There is not enough space here for full discussion of these questions, so we refer to the literature.

*Fig. 15-66*

*Infiltrating lobular carcinoma Special type: Fechner type.* This is another example. Left: Lcis in ducts and in close connection with lobular atypia (arrow in upper part).

Center: Lcis in close connection with infiltrating strands, many of them rather narrow.

Right: Peripheral zone of the tumor showing infiltration in rather broad columns out into the fatty tissue. The cells in the columns are small and regular as usual in lobular carcinomas. This together with Lcis justifies the diagnosis.

This type has been specially described by Fechner.

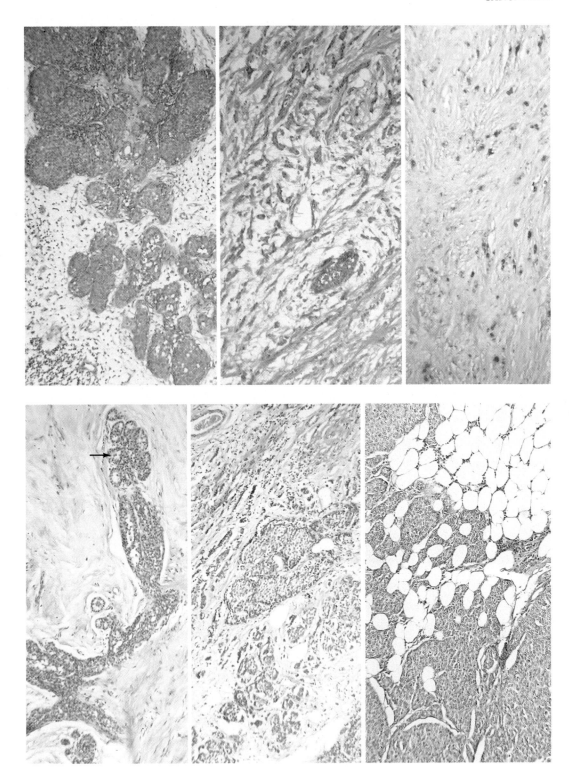

*Fig. 15-67*

*Infiltrating lobular carcinoma Special type? Signet ring cell carcinoma.* This is a very controversial variant. Some pathologists feel that it is lobular carcinoma, while others assert that it is a special carcinoma with no connection to lobular carcinoma. Some carcinomas which infiltrate in narrow rows contain many mucin drops and in common stainings the tumor cells seem vacuolated like signet ring cells. Another name for this type of carcinoma is *epitheliome à cellules, independentes et secretantes.*

This type of tumor is rather rare. We have no definite opinion about the nature of this type and refer to the literature.

Left: Growth in ducts of compact formations of cells many of which contain mucin drops.

Right: A duct surrounded by small infiltrating narrow strands of carcinoma cells.

This type of carcinoma is said to have a less favorable prognosis but large, well defined materials are lacking.

*Fig. 15-68*

*Infiltrating lobular carcinoma. Special type? Signet ring cell carcinoma.* This is another example of this type. Left: Infiltration of light stained cells. They are also seen as small nests in the epithelium.

Right: A detail showing the diffuse infiltration in a loose stroma and a nest of carcinoma cells in the epithelium. The signet ring cell character is obvious. The tumor cells are larger and more atypical than in usual lobular carcinoma. This is not a real Paget lesion (Ch. 17), which is characteristically composed of comedo carcinoma in the milk ducts and large light cells growing diffusely in the epithelium.

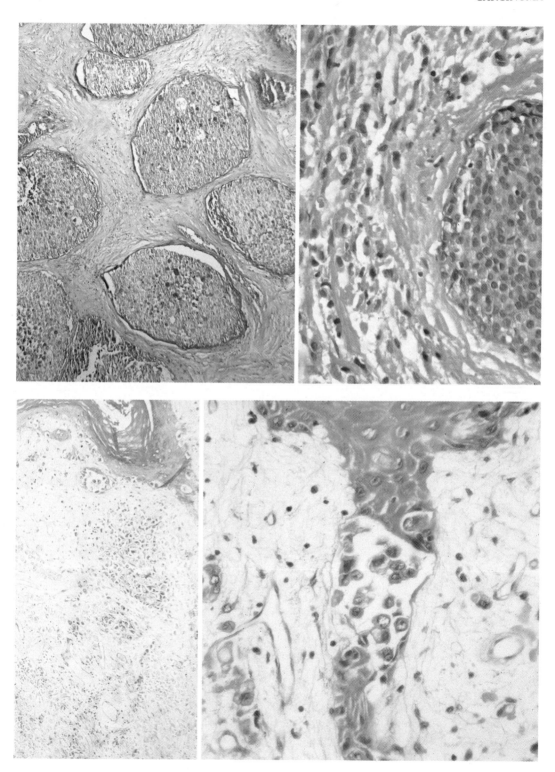

*Fig. 15-69*

*Infiltrating lobular? carcinoma. Signet ring cell carcinoma.* This is another case.

Left: Infiltrating "Indian files" of cells, which are larger than normal in lobular carcinoma. They encircle a duct with normal two-layered epithelium.

Right: A detail showing rather large carcinoma cells with light cytoplasm. In one of the ducts (arrow) the normal two-layered cells are mixed with large light carcinoma cells, a phenomenon which we designate "pagetoid growth".

*Fig. 15-70*

*"Tubulolobular cancer".* This designation was introduced by Fisher et al. (1977) and applied to tumors inbetween lobular and tubular carcinomas. Azzopardi (1979) also depicts such carcinomas as variants of lobular invasive carcinoma. We (Linell et al., 1980) have discussed these problems and have agreed that these carcinomas could be tubular carcinomas progressing to less differentiated tubuloductal carcinomas. This question is open for discussion and we cannot deny the possibility that there exist carcinomas that may fit in with the descriptions of tubulolobular carcinoma. A case which may belong to this category is described here.

This was a 44-year-old woman with a diffuse and uncharacteristic thickening of the breast tissue. Macroscopically there were no typical signs of carcinoma. Histology revealed multiple tubular carcinomas.

To the left, among several normal lobules of varying size there are foci of tubular carcinoma which look like they come from the centers of lobules.

To the right, one of these foci, showing irregular, angulated tubules. A few of them are compact. See the next picture.

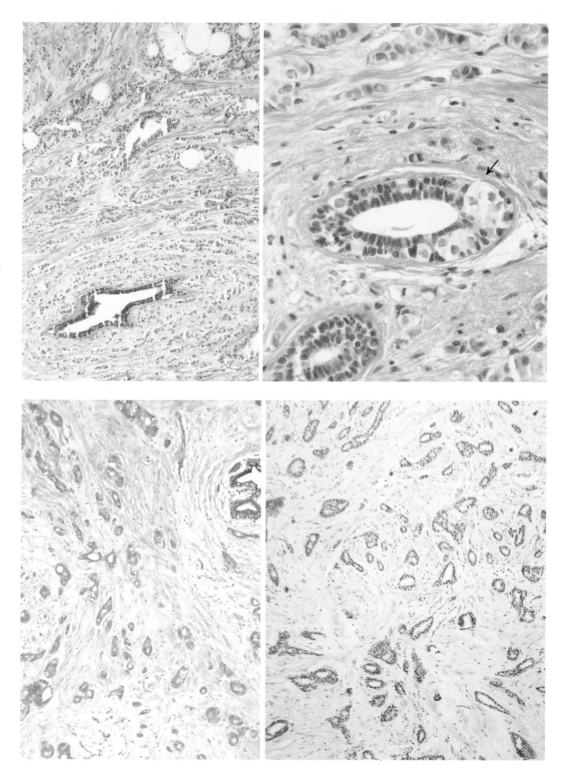

*Fig. 15-71*

*"Tubulolobular carcinoma"*. The same case as in the preceding figure, with elastin staining.

Left: Diffuse growth of tubular carcinoma that seems to be centered around lobules with terminal ducts having thick walls with abundant elastin.

Right: A detail of a tubular carcinoma with cribriform growth in a thick-walled duct with abundant elastin deposits.

The tubular carcinomas in this case are not classic according to the descriptions in Ch. 15. On the other hand we are not convinced that they have any real relation to lobular carcinoma.

We feel that the nature of "tubulolobular" carcinoma must be the object of further research.

In the case here there were no axillary metastases in spite of the diffuse and widespread growth in the breast.

Altogether we have seen two cases of this type.

*Fig. 15-72*

*Adenoid-cystic ccarcinoma*. This cancer type is very rare ( ∼ 0.1%). It has the same histologic appearance as carcinomas with the same name in salivary glands. When occurring in the salivary glands these tumors tend to have a rather sinister prognosis, whereas their mammary counterpart appears to be fairly innocent.

The case shown here is extraordinary in that the tumor had been growing in an old woman for a long time, probably for several years. This is typical of adenoid-cystic carcinomas, which often have a history of 5-6 years.

To the left, the surgical specimen viewed from the outside. A bulky tumor measuring 10×16 cm with an ulceration, 4 cm in diameter. To the right, the cut surface with several lobes of a rather well circumscribed grayish-white medullary tumor. In some places there were hemorrhages and cystic degeneration.

Ten axillary lymph nodes were all free from metastases. After 2 years the patient has had no recurrences.

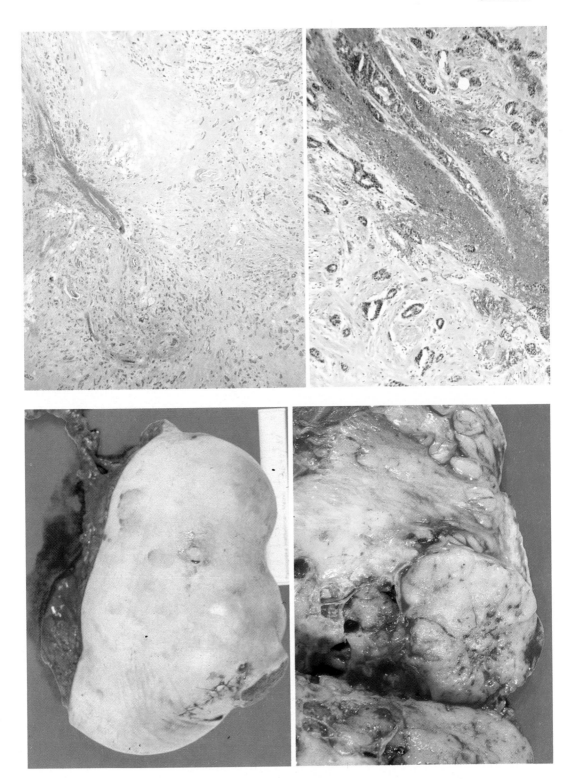

*Fig. 15-73*

*Adenoid-cystic carcinoma.* This carcinoma type has a special histology, which makes it easy to diagnose. It grows in large, rather well deliminated bulky masses, composed of rather uniform middle-sized cells with vesicular nuclei. In the cell masses there are round spaces filled with acid mucin. Azzopardi (1979) has emphasized a dimorphic pattern with ducts differing from other large mucin-filled spaces situated in diffuse proliferations of cells without special arrangements. This dimorphic pattern, which will be presented in the next picture, is essential for differentiating adenoid-cystic carcinoma from cases of cribriform intraductal carcinoma.

To the left, an overview of the tumor with the mucin-filled channels traversing the tumor mass. In the middle, an Alcian-blue-PAS staining, showing the blue acid mucin. To the right, the tumor with a well delimitated border. The cells are uniform with vesicular nuclei and rather small nucleoli.

*Fig. 15-74*

*Adenoid-cystic carcinoma.* This is a further illustration from another case in order to show the typical features. The lobes of the tumor are separated by thin strands of loose connective tissue. The lobes are extremely well delimitated and often angulated.

To the right, the same in more detail. The cells are very uniform. Several mitoses are seen. The "dimorphic pattern" is illustrated by some small ducts (arrows) with palisading cells in contrast to the large mucin-filled channels in the cell masses without special arrangements of the cells around the spaces.

With strict definitions adenoid-cystic cancer is extremely rare (about 0,1%).

Adenoid-cystic carcinoma has a very good prognosis and few cases of generalized spread are known.

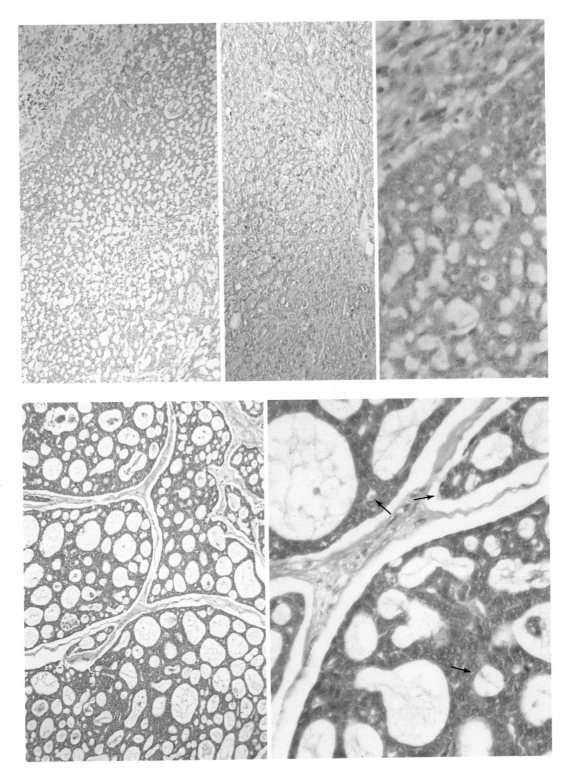

*Fig. 15-75*

*Secretory carcinoma (infantile carcinoma).* This is an extremely rare type of carcinoma. At first it was believed to exist only in children, hence the name *infantile carcinoma*, but several cases in adult young women have now been seen.

The prognosis has been found to be excellent. Later it was realized that this carcinoma type could also be found in adults and because of its pronounced signs of secretion it was named *secretory carcinoma*. It is characterized by lobes composed of large, often vacuolated cells. The cells are often stretched around spaces filled with PAS-positive material.

To the left, an overview showing densely packed cells, often arranged around spaces filled with secretions.

To the right, at a higher magnification. The cells show little atypia and mitoses are very rare. Secretion is sometimes seen intracellularly but most often in lumina, lined by cells.

Only a few secretory carcinomas described have had axillary metastases. At least one case of death from metastases has been reported (Tavassoli & Norris, 1980).

*Fig. 15-76*

*Lipid-rich carcinoma.* This type of carcinoma is rather ill-defined. It consists of large vacuolated or finely granular cells, which contain varying amounts of fat, well visualized in common fat stains.

The cells are arranged in strands separated by narrow streaks often infiltrated by inflammatory cells. Lipid-rich carcinomas are rare, little is known about their prognosis. There are reasons to believe that some of these carcinomas are hidden in the group medullary carcinoma with lymphoid stroma infiltration.

To the left, the compact tumor with light stained cells. To the right, at a high magnification, large amount of vacuolated cytoplasm of the cells. The cells contained large amounts of Oil Red positive material.

The tumor was first described by Aboumrad et al. (1963), who called it "lipid secreting carcinoma" to emphasize that the lipid was not a result of degeneration of the cells. We prefer the more neutral term "lipid-rich". It has been suspected that about 1% of breast carcinomas are lipid-rich. A more frequent use of fat-staining would probably reveal more cases.

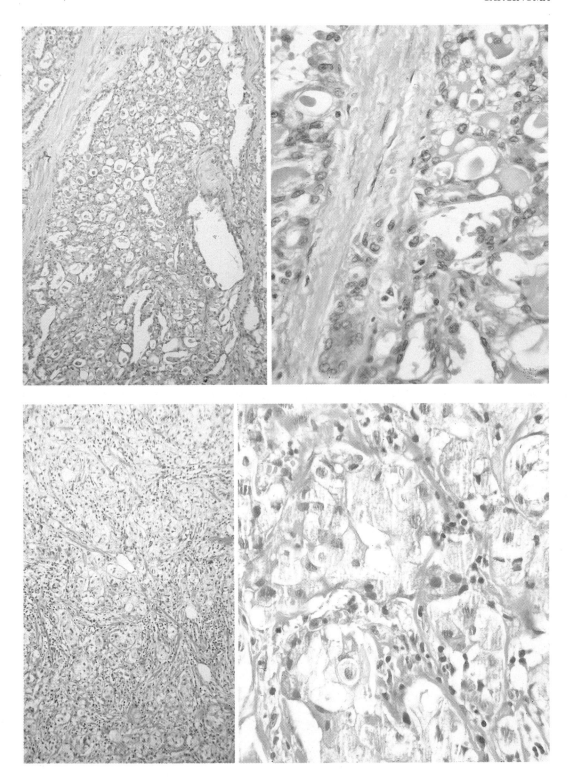

*Fig. 15-77*

*Lipid-rich carcinoma.* The pictures are from the same case. To the left, carcinoma cells in the lower part and at the top a heavy infiltrate of lymphocytes and plasma cells. To the right, an Alcian-blue-PAS staining showing acid muco-substances among the carcinoma cells and sometimes even a few mucin drops in the cytoplasm of the cells. Fat-staining showed both diffuse and drop-like inclusions of fat. The small content of muco-substances alone cannot explain the light color of the cytoplasm in hematoxylin-eosin stainings.

Except for the fat in the cells these carcinomas do not show any special features. One may find medullary carcinomas with the same histologic picture with large, light granular cells but without fat. There are therefore reasons to believe that lipid-rich carcinoma is only a variant of medullary carcinoma with lymphoid stromal infiltration.

The fact that lipid-rich carcinoma has been combined with Paget's nipple disease supports our opinion that it is closely related to carcinoma of comedo type. Further studies may show if there are reasons to classify them as a separate entity.

*Fig. 15-78*

*Carcinoma with giant cells.* Giant cells in carcinomas is a rare finding without known causes or importance. The patient in this case had at least 6 different carcinomas in both breasts. In two of them there were plenty of giant cells of the osteoclast-type.

To the left, picture of the carcinoma made up of glandular structures with tall epithelium. We have interpreted the tumor as an infiltrating comedo carcinoma with glandular structures (cf. Fig. 15 – 38-39).

To the right, many giant cells in the loose cellular stroma surrounding the atypical gland-like structures. Giant cells can also be seen without direct relation to carcinoma in breasts both with and without carcinoma (Rosen, 1979).

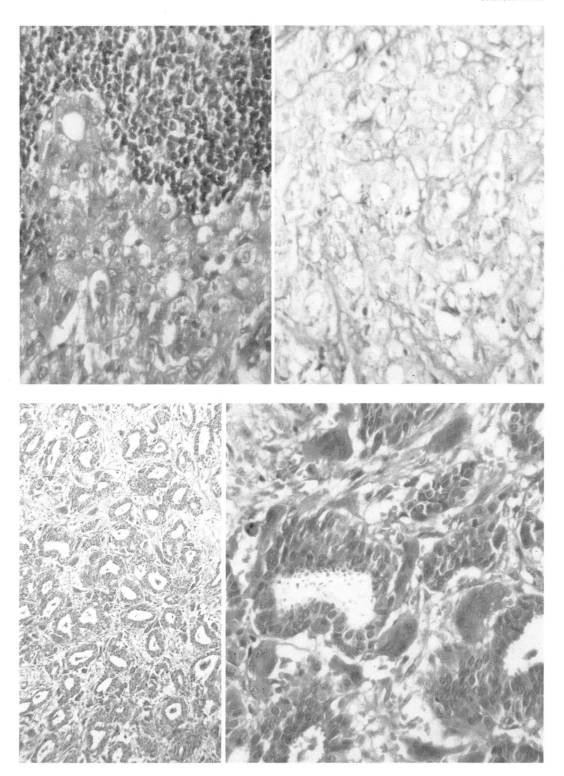

*Fig. 15-79*

*Metaplastic carcinoma (carcinosarcoma)*. Carcinomas of this type are rare findings in the breast as they are in other organs and they always cause difficulties in classification. Due to their rarity we do not know much about their biologic characteristics and prognosis.

To the left, a view of a carcinoma with atypical gland-like structures growing among a diffuse cellular arrangement mimicking a sarcoma.

To the right, large, highly atypical cells in a sarcoma-like pattern. Some of the cells are multinucleated giant cells. There are also some eosinophil islands made up of squamous cell carcinoma.

Tumors of this type have sometimes been called carcinosarcomas. This name ought to be reserved for cases with both epithelial and mesenchymal elements. Cf. Ch. 18. In metaplastic carcinomas we have reason to believe that the sarcoma-like parts are metaplastic epithelial cells.

*Fig. 15-80*

*Breast carcinoma with argyrophil cells – carcinoid tumor?* Breast carcinomas may sometimes contain argyrophil cells in varying proportions. Such cells have been found in the common types of breast carcinoma, most frequently in mucinous carcinomas. Although there have been occasional reports of breast tumors with argyrophil cells which claim that these represent true carcinoid tumors, the majority of breast carcinomas containing such cells appear to have more in common with the conventional breast cancer forms, and should be regarded as distinct from carcinoid tumors. The nature of the argyrophil material in breast carcinomas is obscure. Secretory granules resembling granules in endocrine polypeptide producing cells have been reported on electron microscopy of these cells, but so far no known hormonal peptides have been identified in the cells. Recently immunocytochemical evidence has been found for the presence of lactalbumin in argyrophil cells in breast carcinomas, which may account for the argyrophil reaction in some of these tumors. On the other hand, the high incidence of argyrophil cells in mucinous carcinomas may point to a possible relationship with the production of mucin in these tumors.

This case illustrates a breast carcinoma with argyrophil cells. By hematoxylin-eosin it would be classified as an infiltrating carcinoma of comedo type. Due to a considerable admixture of lymphoid cells in the stroma, in the marginal parts of the tumor it may be included within the subgroup of "medullary carcinoma with lymphoid stroma infiltration". The tumor is very cellular, made up of compact nests of polyhedric atypical cells, bearing no special resemblance to carcinoid tumor cells.

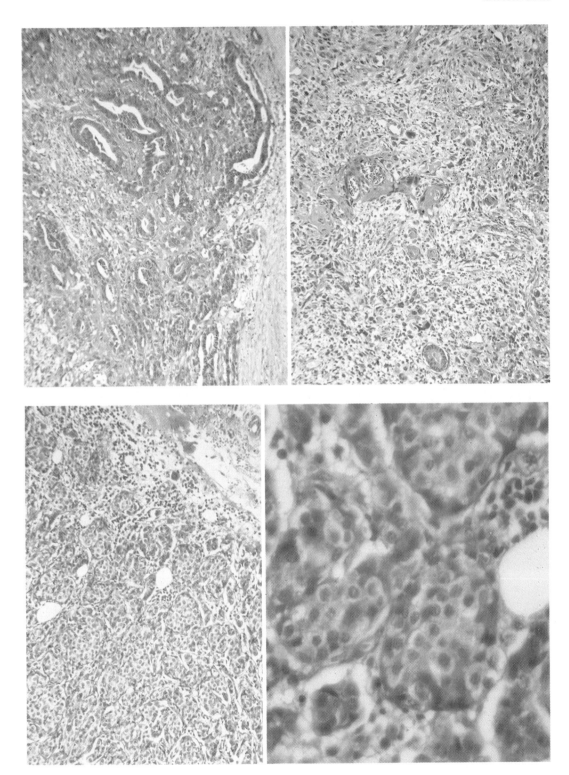

*Fig. 15-81*

*Breast carcinoma with argyrophil cells – carcinoid tumor?* The picture to the left shows argyrophil cells scattered in the nests of tumor cells (Grimelius silver nitrate procedure). The picture to the right shows intracellular mucin, stained with Alcian-blue-PAS. The similarity between the distribution and morphology of the argyrophil material and that of the mucin is very striking, strengthening our belief that in some tumors with argyrophil cells, the argyrophil reaction may be related to the production of mucin.

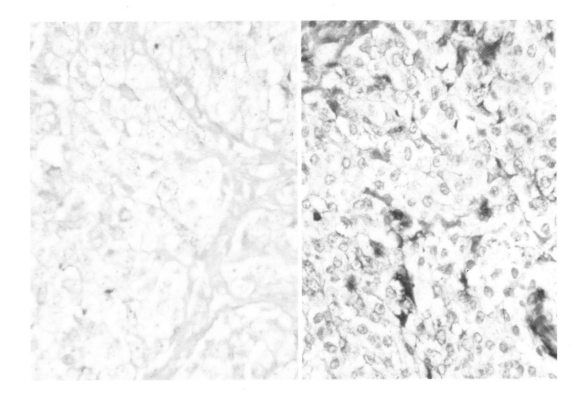

*Fig. 15-82*

*Combined carcinomas (Intraductal comedo carcinoma combined with lobular carcinoma).* Some carcinomas are difficult to classify because they seem to be made up of two different types, each with a typical appearance (Rosen, 1980; Linell et al., 1980). Lobular carcinoma is most often seen together with other carcinomas.

It is well known that carcinomas of different types are seen in one and the same breast (Linell et al., 1980; Ringberg et al., 1982). With this in mind it is reasonable to assume that the two carcinomas may just happen to grow in the same place.

To the left, two ducts filled with cribriform atypical proliferations like a classic intraductal carcinoma with large polymorphous cells. In the surroundings infiltration of "Indian files" of small lobular carcinoma cells and in the lower field a lobular carcinoma in situ (arrow).

To the right, a higher magnification showing the contrast between the large cells of the intraductal carcinoma and the small infiltrating cells of the lobular carcinoma.

*Fig. 15-83*

*Combined carcinomas (Lobular carcinoma combined with intraductal carcinoma or tubular carcinoma).* Left: Three ducts with polymorphous large cells from a comedo carcinoma and single rows of infiltrating lobular carcinoma.

Right: Another case with infiltrating lobular carcinoma in the upper field. At the bottom, infiltrating tubules from a tubular carcinoma. Tubular carcinomas start in radial scars. In the radial scar there are often ducts with epithelial proliferations from which comedo carcinomas may start. It is therefore reasonable to believe that combinations of comedo carcinoma and tubuloductal carcinoma may occasionally appear (Fig. 15-84).

Combined carcinomas are also found in Figs. 15 – 86-87.

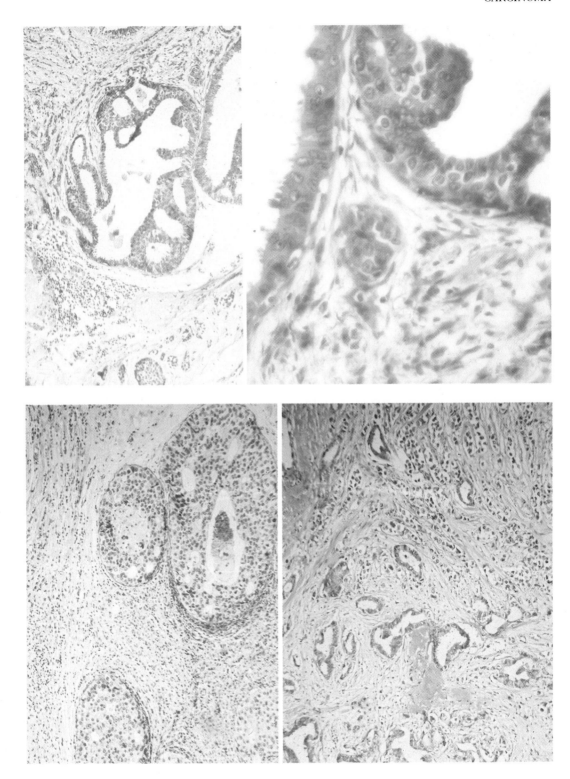

*Fig. 15-84*

*Combined carcinomas (Tubuloductal carcinoma combined with comedo carcinoma)*. This is the most common combination, which is quite natural as we regard combined carcinomas as fortuitous developments of 2 carcinomas in the immediate vicinity of each other. There would be the greatest chance of this happening with the two most common types of carcinoma.

Left: In the upper field, a papillary intraductal carcinoma with a sharp border on a tubular carcinoma. Center: The tubular carcinoma at higher magnification. Right: The part containing intraductal comedo carcinoma. In this case it is easy to see that there are *two* different carcinomas, but in other instances, as for example when a tubular carcinoma + or 0 is combined with an intraductal and infiltrating comedo carcinoma, there can be difficulties in interpretation.

Such cases may also cause difficulties in classification and in assessing the prognostic factors.

*Fig. 15-85*

*Bilateral carcinoma*. Several reports indicate that meticulous studies of mastectomy specimens besides the study carcinoma may also reveal other multiple invasive or *in situ* carcinomas in up to 65-75% of the cases (for references, see Linell et al., 1980).

It is natural to think that there are many carcinomas in the contralateral breast. Space does not permit a more detailed discussion of this problem and we refer to Ringberg et al. (1982) for more references.

The picture shows an example of bilateral carcinoma. To the left, the first carcinoma (a comedo carcinoma with mucin production) in a 43-year-old woman. Seven years later a reconstruction of the breast was made and at the same time a subcutaneous mastectomy done on the other side. The specimen was totally embedded and sectioned and in *one* section the small intraductal carcinoma was found (seen in the picture on the right). This was an incidental finding. If a total sectioning had not been performed, the small lesion would probably not have been found. With this method we have found carcinomas in the contralateral breast in about 45% of the cases of bilateral subcutaneous mastectomy. This high figure supports the view that many of these small tumors remain quiescent or even regress. But we do not know how to distinguish these tumors from those which are aggressive and will cause a clinically malignant disease.

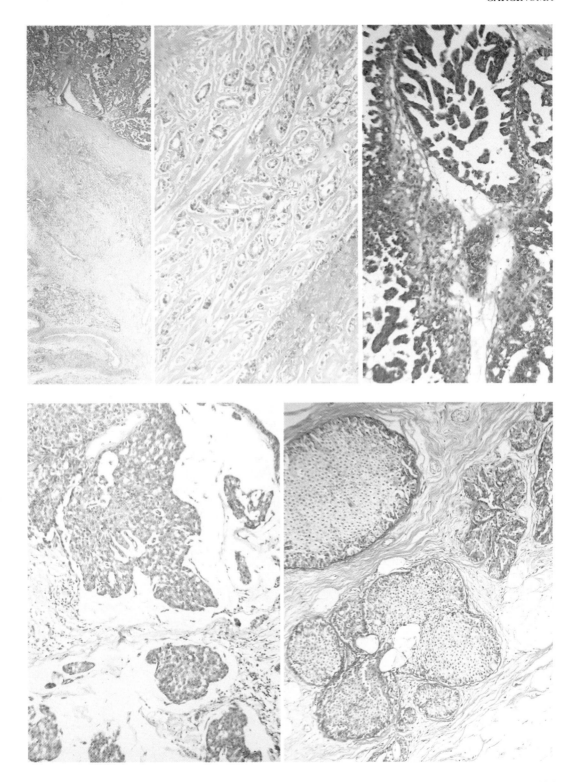

*Fig. 15-86*

*"Occult carcinoma"*. The case, showed in this and the following pictures, can be said to illustrate *occult carcinoma* as well as *combined carcinoma* and *bilateral carcinoma*.

The 48-year-old patient had a monozygote twin, who had had a tubuloductal carcinoma 3 years previously and underwent a reconstruction operation and at the same time a contralateral reduction plasty. The specimen showed lobular carcinoma in situ. A subcutaneous mastectomy was then performed and this specimen showed large numbers of lobular in situ carcinomas. These findings made her twin sister seek her doctor, who, considering her a risk case, advised a bilateral subcutaneous mastectomy. Her breasts were subjectively, clinically and mammographically normal. Both specimens were extensively sectioned and showed in about half of the slides numerous foci of both ductal and lobular in situ carcinomas, illustrated here.

To the left, a field filled with typical lobular carcinoma in situ and to the right, intraductal carcinoma of comedo type, comprising rather large cells in cribriform and bridging structures.

*Fig. 15-87*

*"Occult" carcinoma*. Same case as in the foregoing picture. T the left, a field with lobular carcinoma in situ in lower part and intraductal comedo carcinoma with cancerization of lobules (arrows).

To the right, a dilated duct surrounded by lobular carcinoma in situ. The duct shows a micropapillary intraductal carcinoma with large cells. The cores of the papillae are made up of small cells from lobular carcinoma in situ.

This case is of great interest, showing a widespread bilateral carcinoma in situ without any symptoms.

At the same time it gives rise to some reflections on hereditary breast carcinoma. In these two monozygote twins there is strong reason to believe that genetic factors have played a large role in cancerogenesis. The two twins had altogether 3 types of carcinoma: tubuloductal carcinoma, lobular carcinoma and ductal comedo carcinoma of several subtypes.

The findings in this case suggest that genetic factors are not bound to produce a special histologic type of carcinoma, but seem to exert a carcinogenic action that can result in different histologic types of carcinoma.

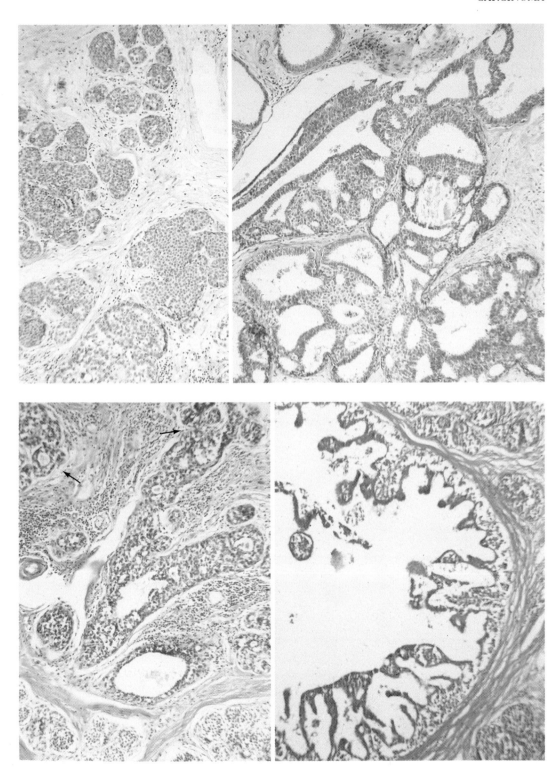

*Fig. 15-88*

*"Regressing" carcinoma.* This is a very controversial theme. By 1941 Muir had already described two cases of intraductal comedo carcinoma, which he interpreted as regressing carcinoma with necrosis and inflammation. A similar case was described by Linell et al. (1980). Here we show similar pictures from a mural (clinging) carcinoma.

Left: A conglomerate of dilated ducts with thick hyalinized walls. Most of them have no epithelium but in the upper part there is a duct (arrow) with preserved, very dark epithelium and a round cell infiltrate in the vicinity.

Center: In the upper field, an obliterated duct (arrow) with wrinkled walls. In the lower part, a duct with regular epithelium.

Right: A duct with thick, bridging, highly atypical epithelium of a cancerous nature. In this case, ducts devoid of epithelium may suggest a desquamation and destroying of the carcinoma. But as in other such cases we will never know if the destruction was complete. On the other hand we can only diagnose carcinoma if some of it is preserved. The controversial problem of regression of carcinoma seems to be impossible to solve.

*Fig. 15-89*

*"Regressing" carcinoma.* Intraductal comedo carcinoma with signs of spontaneous regression.

Left: A group of ducts with thick fibrous walls surrounded by sleeves of round cells. Some of the ducts contain necrotic calcified cells but others show cancerous proliferations in the lumen (arrow).

Right: In the center the arrow-marked duct with polymorphous intraductal carcinoma. In the duct wall heavy infiltration with round cells, but in one place (arrow) there is calcified material, probably necrotic carcinoma cells. See Fig. 15-90.

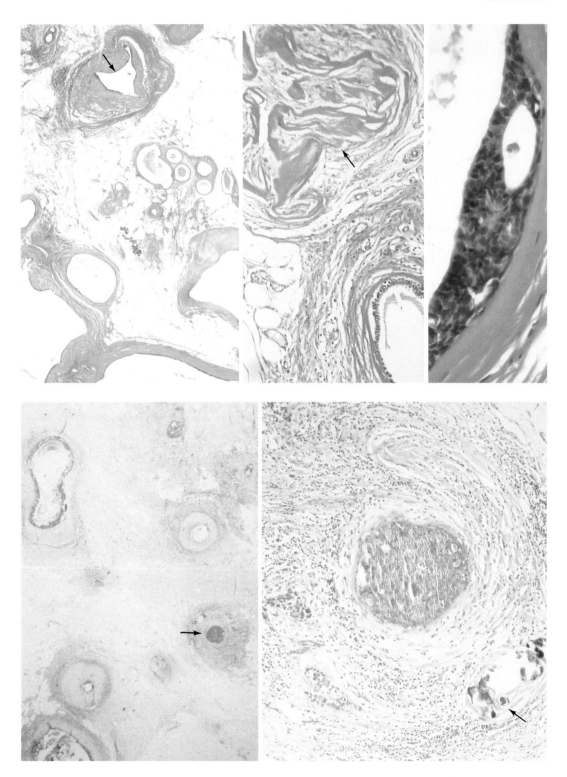

*Fig. 15-90*

*"Regressing" carcinoma.* This is from the same case as in Fig. 15-89.

Left: Ducts with arrows show both calcified material and viable cancerous growth. Another duct (double arrow) shows only calcified material.

Right: A thick-walled duct with a thick mantle of round cells. In the lumen, necrotic debris. Such cases with extensive necrosis in intraductal comedo carcinoma are very suggestive of a spontaneous healing, but it is only (see text to Fig. 15-88) when we see vital cancer cells that we can be certain of the diagnosis.

Muir & Aitkenhead (1934) reported two such cases. They are not uncommon.

*Fig. 15-91*

*Ductectasia with elastosis (Regressed carcinoma?)* Besides the elastosis seen in radial scars and tubuloductal carcinomas, elastosis can also be seen in and around duct walls. (For references see Lundmark 1972 and Azzopardi et al. Ch. 14).

To the left, a dilated duct with some debris in the lumen. The wall is composed of acellular connective tissue and around the duct there are abundant elastin deposits.

To the right, part of the same duct at higher magnification. This type of elastosis was thought by Jackson & Orr (1957) to be "precancerous", an idea rejected by Azzopardi. It might, however, conceivably be postcancerous.

Pictures like this can also be seen in a case as that depicted in Figs. 15 – 88-89. One could therefore hypothesize that the pictures in Fig. 15-91 represent remnants of a totally regressed carcinoma. This hypothesis awaits further studies.

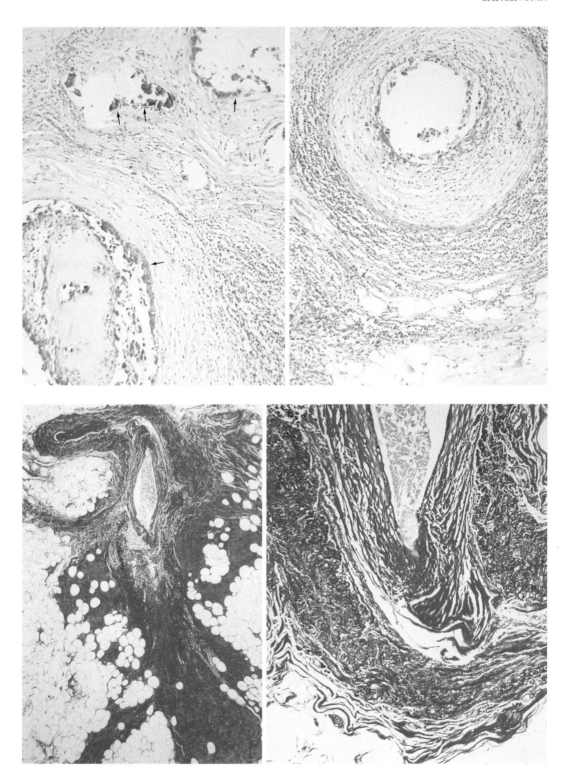

*Fig. 15-92*

*Tubular carcinoma in regression?* This is a curious case from a 71-year-old woman who had a large tumor that mammographically and macroscopically was a typical star-shaped tubuloductal carcinoma. Microscopically, there was a 3 mm hyalin structure in the center (arrow), probably an obliterated duct. Beneath it (arrows) a small, about 1 mm typical tubular carcinoma better seen in the picture on the right. The main part of the spiculated tumor consisted of a granulation tissue filling most of the picture on the left. This granulation tissue is illustrated in more detail in the next figure.

*Fig. 15-93*

*Tubular carcinoma in regression?* Left: In the upper part, a small piece of the tubular carcinoma and in the lower part, granulation tissue with proliferation of fibroblasts. There are also several strands that mimic giant cells. These are better seen in the middle picture and have been interpreted as capillary sprouts. Right: Another part of the inflammatory process with an infiltrate of plasma cells and lymphocytes surrounding a duct.

We have interpreted this as a case of regression of a tubular carcinoma because of the small remnant of carcinoma centrally and the star-shape of the granulation tissue. It is the only case we have seen and our interpretation is purely hypothetical and only made to arouse interest in others in finding additional such cases.

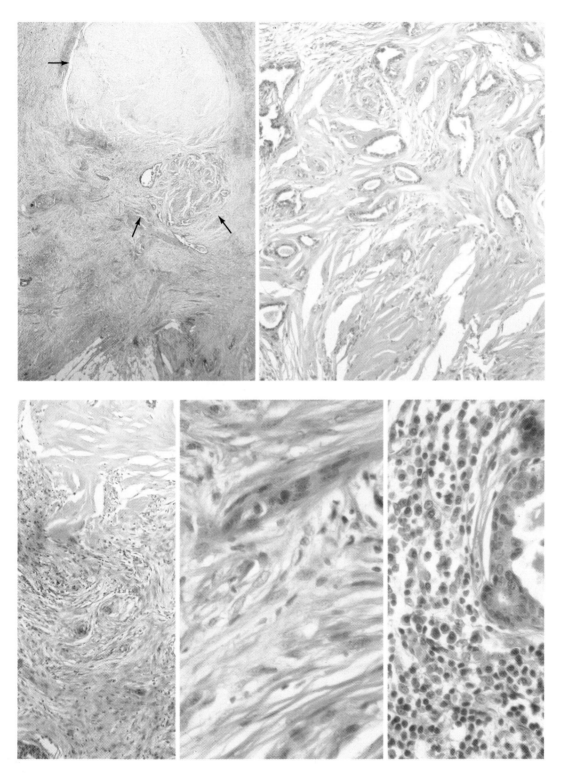

*Fig. 15-94*

*"Intraductal" growth in lymph node metastasis.* This is a rather common finding in comedo carcinoma. The picture shows two fields from a lymph node metastasis. Against a background of diffusely growing carcinoma, several well demarcated round cancer columns with central necroses. The picture exactly mimics intraductal growth.

This is impossible in a lymph node and the explanation must be growth in lymphatic vessels. The importance of this finding has been pointed out by Cowen.

We thought earlier that this type of growth in the breast was always intraductal and proof of the primary carcinoma in that area. This idea must be revised as this type of "intraductal" growth in the breast may possibly be metastatic. The finding is also interesting in the light of Ozello's electron microscopic findings that light-microscopic intraductal growth is not always strictly intraductal and may explain the rare cases where we find metastases when only "intraductal growth" is found in the breast.

*Fig. 15-95*

*"Intraductal" growth of tubular carcinoma outside the breast.* This is a case of tubular carcinoma. Besides infiltrating tubules, cribriform growth in dilated spaces is also seen. The picture mimics the intraductal growth in tubular carcinoma, but in this case the carcinoma grows in the fascia and muscle in an area without breast tissue and the growth is probably located in lymph vessels. This is also something to consider in our common interpretation of "intraductal" growth in tubular carcinomas.

The cases shown here have certainly a general implication for the growth of carcinomas in many other parts of the body.

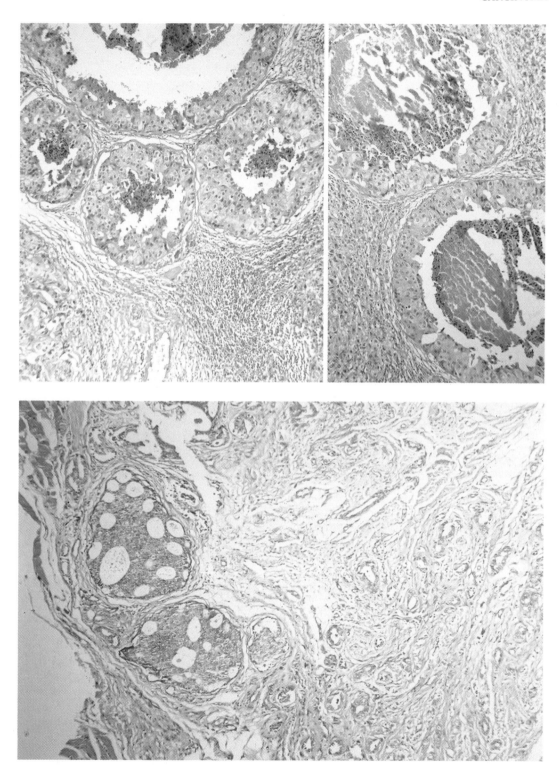

*Fig. 15-96*

*Atypical metastases of lobular carcinoma.* Lymph node metastases of lobular carcinoma have a very characteristic growth manner in lymph nodes, often growing as a lymphoma. This lymphoma-like growth in lymph nodes is very helpful for the diagnosis of lobular carcinoma. The figure here shows a rather rare type of growth. Left: Picture of a lymph node. At both ends there is diffuse lymphoma-like growth, but in the middle part there is growth in rounded formations. Center and right: These formations more clearly shown. They are rounded, well demarcated, look amazingly like the compact end-tubules of lobule, filled with cells as in a lobular carcinoma in situ. This is probably also an example of growth in lymph vessels. In the lower part, the lymphoma-like growth pattern.

*Fig. 15-97*

*Elastin production in a lymph node metastasis from a tubuloductal carcinoma.* Left: View of a small lymph node totally occupied by metastasis. There is also periglandular tumor growth. In the center of the lymph node there are abundant deposits of elastin. Right: At higher magnification. Such elastin deposits are very rarely seen in carcinoma metastasis but contribute to the discussion of how elastin is formed. Probably, the metastatic tumor cells elicit elastin production and they are possibly related to those cells constituting the central tubules in radial scars (Ch. 14).

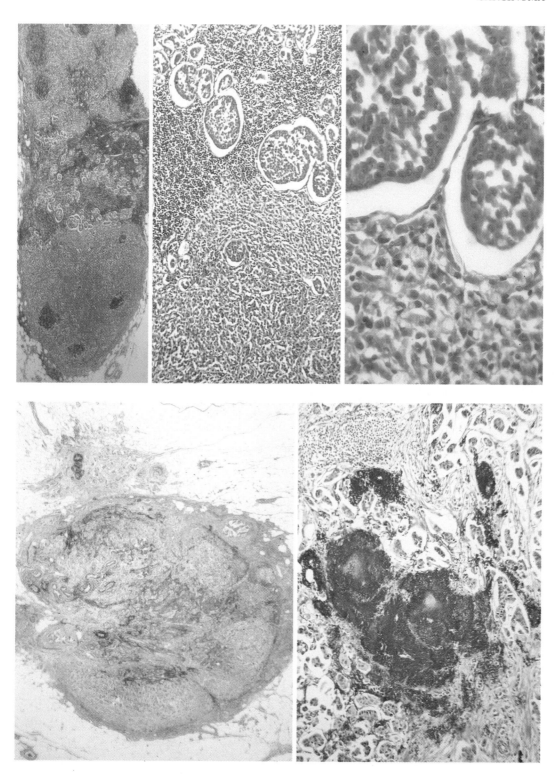

*Chapter 16*

# Mesenchymal Tumors

*Fig. 16-1*

*Cystosarcoma phyllodes.* This tumor represents a very difficult and controversial problem. The name is one of the oldest in tumor pathology, coined already by Johannes Müller in 1838, the teacher of Virchow. The name implies that it was understood to be a malignant tumor. Later on it was found that many of these tumors behaved in a benign manner. It has been proposed that they should be called *giant fibroadenoma.* This is not a good name because these tumors are certainly not fibroadenomas and, nevertheless, some of them are malignant and metastasize. They can show wide variations in histologic structure. We will illustrate some types in the following pictures.

The figure shows the breast of a 37-year-old woman who had noticed a large tumor in one breast. Mammographically it was a well demarcated tumor 10 cm in size. A subcutaneous mastectomy was performed and the figure shows the tumor after opening of a cyst containing many papillary structures, which were edematous.

*Fig. 16-2*

*Cystosarcoma phyllodes.* The tumors often seem to be contained in a cyst and the papillary projection can be divided in leaf-like structures ("blätterige Aufsplitterung"), the origin of the name "phyllodes tumor", (phyllox = leaf). In the upper part, the outer limit as a thin cyst wall. The papillary projections are covered with mostly regular one- or two-layered epithelium. The tumors have no real capsule. Right: Details with a very cellular stroma with atypia and often with many mitoses. The dilemma is that we cannot predict the outcome. In most cases a radical extirpation (local or by mastectomy) will result in a benign course but in some cases distant metastases (mostly in the lung) will appear, often after several years. The metastases are pure sarcomas. Lymph node metastases are very seldom seen. Local excision may be followed by a high incidence of local recurrences.

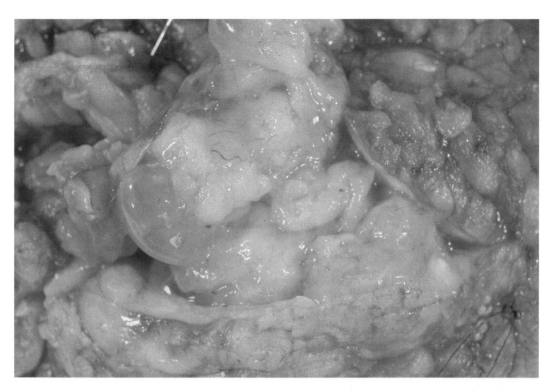

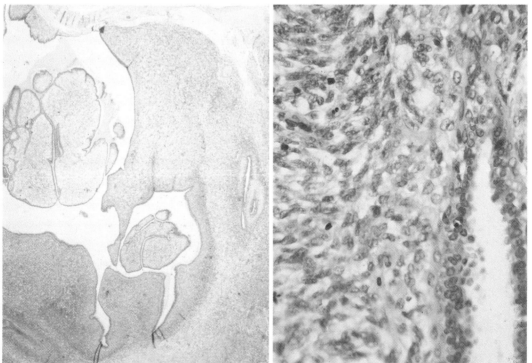

*Fig. 16-3*

*Cystosarcoma phyllodes.* This is another typical example. To the left, the cystic space with epithelium covering papillary projections. The stroma is very cellular but not especially atypical and mitoses are few (picture on the right). In this case the chance for a benign course would appear to be very good, but the course is in reality unpredictable. Cystosarcoma phyllodes shows different pictures in different parts. The stroma may be partly very cellular and in other parts rather acellular and fibrous.

The epithelium is mostly regular and in this case two-layered. When a cystosarcoma metastasizes the epithelium is not involved.

*Fig. 16-4*

*Cystosarcoma phyllodes.* This case is interesting because it illustrates the growth and propagation of these tumors.

In the picture to the left the tumor is divided in several parts. At least three cysts show up with papillary infoldings. These three parts have no capsules. The stroma is moderately cellular.

To the right, several "sub-tumors" of the same type. They seem to grow in lobules in the vicinity of the large tumor. This is certainly not an outgrowth from the central tumor but an evolution of new tumor. This phenomenon probably explains the tendency for local "recurrences", even after apparently radical local extirpation.

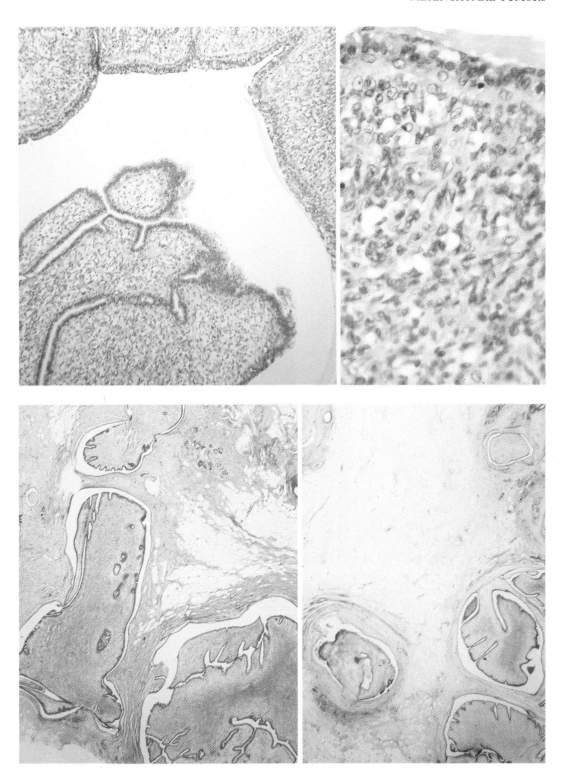

*Fig. 16-5*

*Cystosarcoma phyllodes.* Picture showing the phyllodes character of the tumor and at the same time how ill-demarcated it is. It borders on the surrounding tissue with lobules without the slightest sign of a capsule. In the lower part, the same type of propagation (arrows) as shown in Fig. 16-4.

*Fig. 16-6*

*Cystosarcoma phyllodes with ductal carcinoma in situ.* This was a 37-year-old woman with a mass in the left breast. Fine needle aspiration biopsy showed carcinoma cells. The tumor was gelatinous and appeared well demarcated.

Left: Picture of the tumor. At the lower left, the well demarcated border. The tumor is cellular, with branched clefts of phyllodes type, lined by prominent epithelial masses.

Right: The stroma is cellular with many mitoses. The ducts are partly filled with atypical epithelial masses. The nuclei are large and polymorphous and mitoses are seen. The picture corresponds to intraductal carcinoma of comedo type.

The stroma in this case resembles that in cystosarcoma phyllodes. The epithelium in cystosarcoma phyllodes is mostly benign and this case is very unusual.

The woman was treated with bilateral subcutaneous mastectomy. The specimens were totally sectioned but all showed a normal picture. There were no abnormal epithelial proliferations in other places.

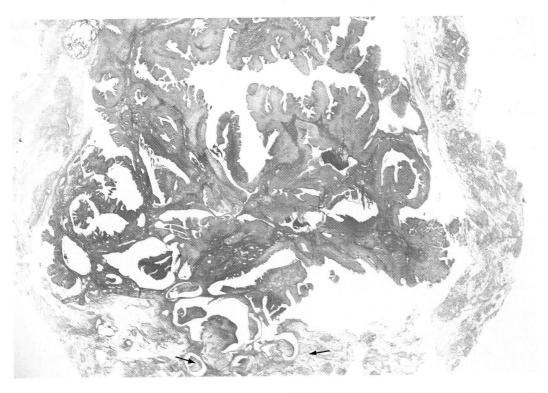

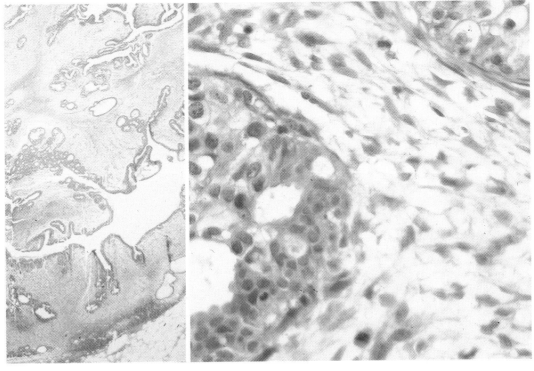

*Fig. 16-7*

*Cystosarcoma phyllodes with metaplastic changes.* Left: Overview of the tumor. On the right in the picture the well demarcated border with round cell infiltration. The architecture of the tumor is in between that of a fibroadenoma and a phyllodes tumor.

The epithelial clefts and islands are very irregularly arranged.

Right: The highly cellular stroma. The epithelial structures often show squamous epithelial metaplasia. They contain vacuoles. Sebaceous gland metaplasia is seen in several places (arrows). Details in the next picture.

*Fig. 16-8*

*Cystosarcoma phyllodes with metaplastic changes.* The picture shows two details of the tumor from the foregoing picture. The stroma is cellular and atypical. The epithelial islands show moderate atypia and, interestingly, a marked cytoplasmic vacuolization. In the picture on the right the cells clearly show sebaceous differentiation.

This case was initially interpreted as a malignant cystosarcoma phyllodes. We do not know the exact biologic nature of the tumor, and can only note that the patient lives without signs of recurrence 10 years after mastectomy.

The cases shown here are used to illustrate that "cystosarcoma phyllodes" is a tumor with many different facets. We have shown rare cases with epithelial neoplasia and metaplasia. The stromal component may also show different metaplastic changes (see Figs. 16 – 9-10).

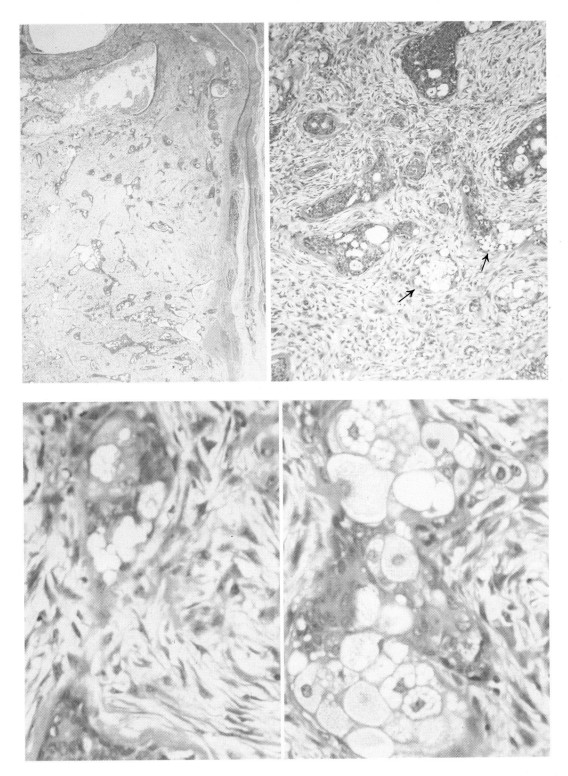

*Fig. 16-9*

*Phyllodes tumor with metaplastic epithelial and sarcomatous features.* This case is a phyllodes tumor with peculiar epithelial and stromal changes.

Left: In the upper part, a cystic space lined by epithelium. Below there are several epithelium lined tubules in a cellular stroma giving the impression of a close relationship to a phyllodes tumor. In the lower part there is a pure sarcomatous pattern, which is seen at a higher magnification in the picture on the right. The tumor resembles a fibrosarcoma with many mitoses.

*Fig. 16-10*

*Phyllodes tumor with metaplastic epithelial and sarcomatous features.* The picture shows details from the foregoing case.

Left: An epithelial island with squamous metaplasia and cornification lying in a sarcoma-like stroma. On the right a cyst with cylindrical epithelium. The stroma is very cellular with atypia.

Right: Another field of the tumor showing a delicate lacework of osteoid trabeculae intermingled with atypical sarcoma cells, a true picture of an osteoblastic sarcoma.

The tumor in this case has some traits pointing to an origin from a phyllodes tumor. Other types of "metaplastic" sarcomas such as lipasarcomas and fibrosarcomas have been reported to occur in phyllodes tumors. In the breast different sarcomas without connection with phyllodes tumors are also encountered. An example of this is to be found in Figs. 16 – 11-12.

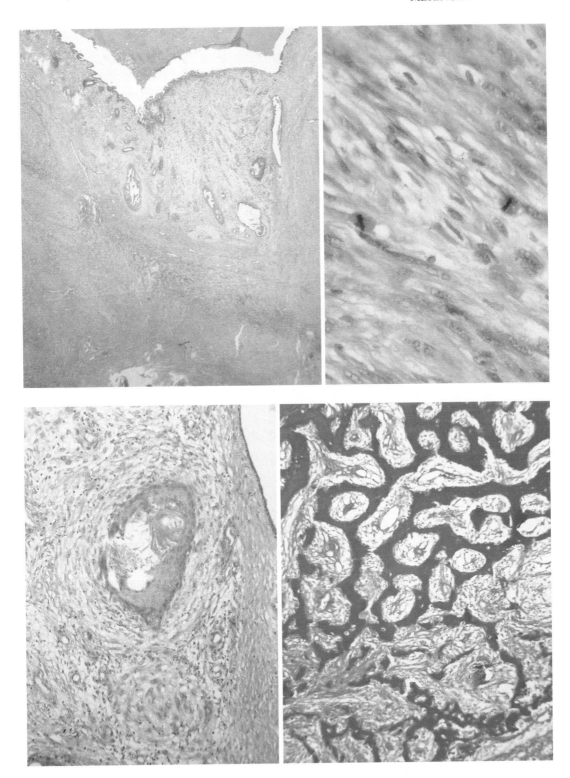

*Fig. 16-11*

*Osteogenic sarcoma.* This case was a 57-year-old woman who presented with a large ulcerated tumor in her right breast. A mastectomy was performed. The picture to the left shows the large tumor, rather well delimited, in the fatty breast tissue. The tumor has a polycyclic border and shows areas of disintegration and cysts. The tumor was an osteogenic sarcoma (the histology is shown in Fig. 16-12). Five years after mastectomy the tumor recurred locally. The picture to the right shows the bulging mass in the thoracic wall. One and a half years later the patient died. Autopsy showed widespread metastases, especially in the lungs.

*Fig. 16-12*

*Osteogenic sarcoma.* Histology of the foregoing case shows a cellular stroma with osteoid tissue, partly calcified.

To the right, a higher magnification with osteoid tissue with large atypical cells in the lacunae. Around the tissue we see the cellular stroma and attempts to form osteoblastic rows on the osteoid trabeculae.

This is an example of a pure sarcoma of the breast. We should probably interpret these sarcomas (fibrosarcoma, liposarcoma, chondrosarcoma, osteosarcoma, myosarcoma, etc.) as common soft tissue sarcomas that happen to arise in the connective tissue of the breasts. They mostly cause no diagnostic troubles.

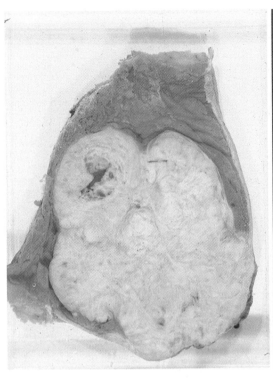
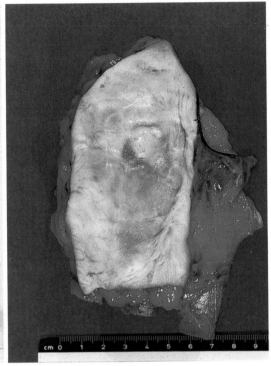
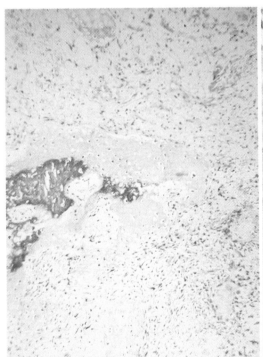
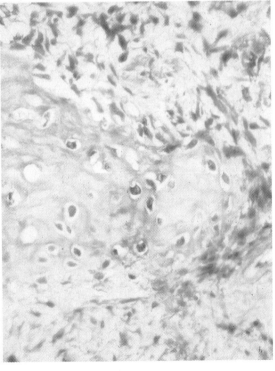

*Fig. 16-13*

*Angioma.* Vascular tumors in the breast are said to be rather rare. Small angiomas which are often restricted to the stroma of a single lobule are easily overlooked and are of no clinical importance. Such an incidental finding is seen here. Among several normal lobules there is a conglomerate of blood-filled spaces in the interlobular connective tissue. The vessel walls are thin and there are no signs of malignancy.

In some benign lesions (hamartoma Ch. 13) there is sometimes a stroma with many vessels but these changes have no neoplastic properties.

*Fig. 16-14*

*Angiosarcoma.* These tumors are rare. They have a rapid course with poor prognosis. They can be found at all ages. They are often bulky tumors with a dark discoloration of the skin. At operation they bleed easily and profusely. Histologically there is a diffuse proliferation of irregular vascular spaces, infiltrating both intra- and interlobular stroma. The tumors are ill-defined. These *hemangiosarcomas* or *hemangioendotheliomas* do not metastasize to the axillary lymph nodes but soon tend to give widespread visceral metastases.

To the left, picture of the haphazardly arranged vascular spaces. To the right, a detail showing the atypical endothelial cells lining spaces with red blood corpuscles. The vessels penetrate between the tubules of a lobule.

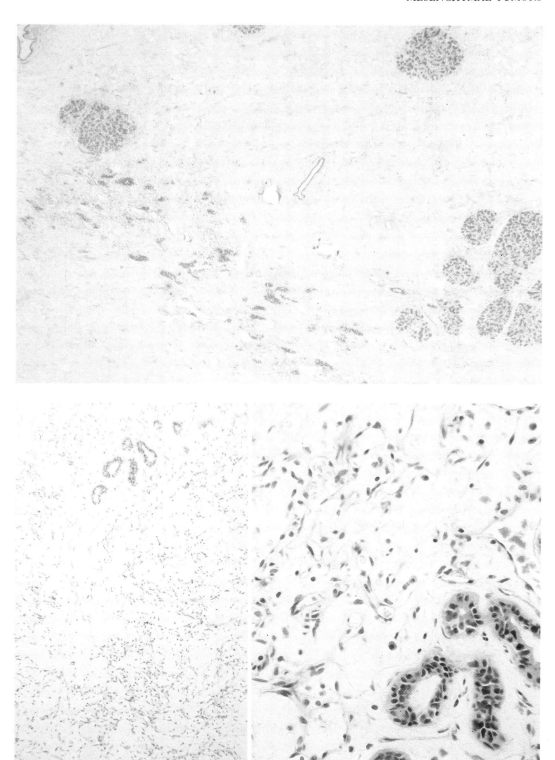

*Fig. 16-15*

*Angiosarcoma*. This is another example. The lobular structures are preserved among the vascular channels. This tumor is more cellular than in the preceding case. The detail to the right shows the anastomosing blood-filled channels very clearly. There is also an atypical cellular proliferation in the tissue in between the open channels.

A vascular tumor with a special connection to the breast is the *hemolymphangiosarcomas seen in Stewart-Treves syndrome*. They are not located in the breast tissue but start in lymphedematous tissue, usually in the arm after a mastectomy with axillary exeresis. They grow and metastasize rapidly. (Because they are generally seen in the extremities they are not illustrated in this book).

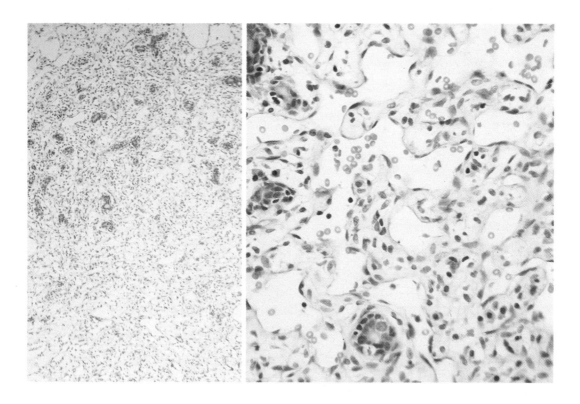

# Chapter 17

# Mammillary Lesions

*Fig. 17-1*

*Paget's nipple disease.* This is the most characteristic nipple disease, which macroscopically appears as an "eczematous" disease on the top of the nipple with serous or bloody discharge and later ulceration. Ever since its description by Paget in 1874 there have been controversial views on this disease. This will be further discussed.

Left: Overview showing the light cells easily visible at low magnification. Center: The light cells are clearly seen. They often show mitoses and have large nuclei with prominent nucleoli.

Right: Field from the transverse section of the mammilla. In the lower part, a normal milk duct but in the upper part, an intraductal carcinoma with pronounced necrosis. To find such an intraductal carcinoma, which is often confined to one or a few of the milk ducts, the transverse section is essential.

Paget's nipple disease can be a localized disease, confined to the nipple, but it may also be part of a generalized comedo carcinoma and is then easily overlooked unless the mammilla is routinely studied.

For many years there have been controversial opinions about Paget's disease. The two most common, diametrically opposite opinions are:
1. The disease starts in the epidermis.
2. The disease starts in the milk ducts and the Paget cells spread secondarily into the epidermis.

It is quite clear that epithelial changes of Paget's type are only seen if we have growth of comedo carcinoma in the milk ducts. If an infiltrating comedo carcinoma grows into the skin from below, outside the mammilla we can get an ulceration but not Paget's disease.

*Fig. 17-2*

*Tubuloductal carcinoma in the mammilla (Invasive ductal carcinoma).* Occasionally we encounter growth of tubuloductal carcinoma in the mammilla. It is characteristic that the carcinoma does not grow in the milk ducts but in the stroma around them. The intraductal component in tubuloductal carcinomas is not as prominent as in comedo carcinoma. The intraductal spread with "cancerization" of lobules is not seen in tubuloductal carcinomas. This must be a profound biological difference.

To the left several ducts with normal epithelial cells. They are encircled by narrow strands of the carcinoma, but we have no growth in the milk ducts.

To the right at two magnifications carcinoma cells are seen invading the epithelium from beneath. This is almost never seen and the picture is different from genuine Paget's disease. The carcinoma cells are smaller and look degenerated and they lie in large vacuoles.

Another change of this type is seen in signet ring cell carcinoma in Fig. 15-68.

260

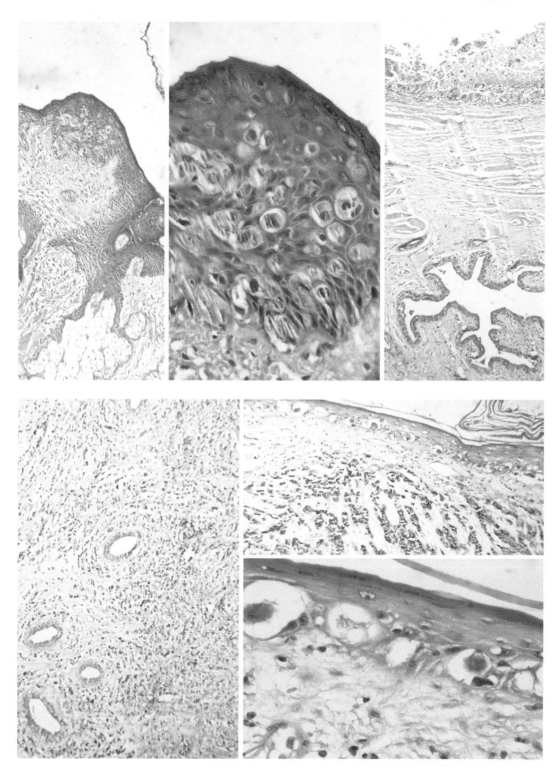

*Fig. 17-3*

*Florid adenomatosis of the mammilla.* This is a rather rare lesion, which because of its site on the mammilla and frequent penetration to the surface is easy to find and diagnose. It was described and named in the beginning of the fifties by Jones.

The symptoms are secretion and bleeding and a fungating tumor will sooner or later appear. The tumor is related to papillary syringocystadenoma of the skin and often shows a papillary pattern on the surface, a feature which may be missed in the sections.

In the picture there is an unaffected epidermis on the surface and no penetration point. The tumor consists of tubules in sclerotic stroma and small cysts filled with papillary excrescences.

For details see next picture.

*Fig. 17-4*

*Florid adenomatosis of the mammilla.* This is the same case as in Fig. 17-3. The two details can easily be found in the foregoing picture: They show papillary folding inwards and adenomatoid structures. The epithelium is one- or two-layered and there is no real atypia. The stroma is rather sclerotic. Such a lesion is considered wholly benign and there are large series in the literature indicating this (see references). In spite of this we often find in the published materials that the pathologist has reported adenocarcinoma and in many cases mastectomy has been done, which usually was certainly unnecessary. But an uncritical, dogmatic assumption of benignity in every case is unjustified as shown in the following examples.

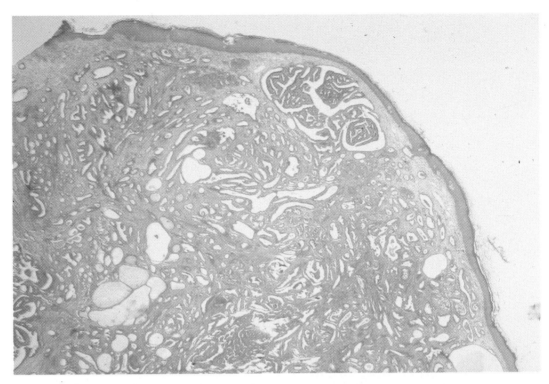

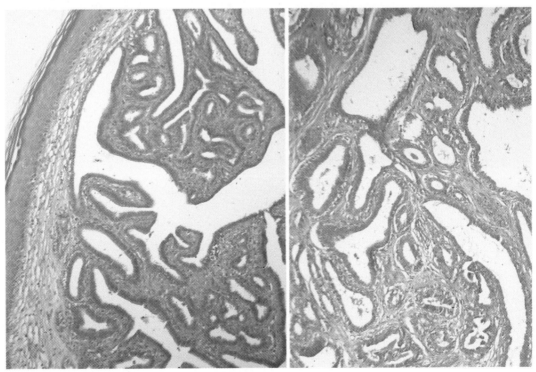

*Fig. 17-5*

*Florid adenomatosis of the mammilla with pronounced atypia.* In this case the mammilla was retracted. At the upper left there is much wrinkling and folding of the skin with a narrow crypt going down to the real mammillary surface. Here we have an opening of the papillary structures on the surface, better seen in the detail on the right. The tubular structures have rather tall and atypical epithelium. In some places two cell layers are discerned.

*Fig. 17-6*

*Florid adenomatosis of the mammilla with pronounced atypia.* These are details from the foregoing case. To the left, tubular structures with tall multi-layered epithelium. In other places there is two-layered epithelium, which has often been taken as proof of its benign nature, especially when the tubules are surrounded by a hyaline stroma, as seen here. This seems to us too dogmatic.

To the right, in detail, the tall atypical epithelium. The cell layers are deranged and there is cellular atypia. A mitosis (arrow) is seen.

We cannot find any clearcut indications of carcinoma but we look upon the case as potentially malignant, based on our experience that long-standing cases of this type have shown metastases. See the following case.

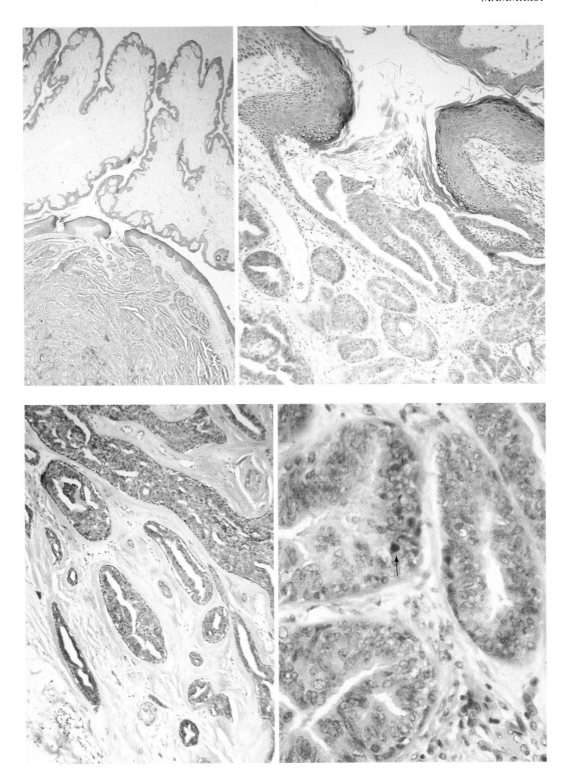

*Fig. 17-7*

*Mammillary adenocarcinoma.* This was a 56-year-old patient who had observed a growing tumor on her right nipple for at least 2-3 years. The tumor was now 2 cm and had an eroded surface.

To the left, surface with many papillary structures showing a wide fungating tumor surface. Beneath this, are densely packed tubular structures.

To the right there are tubular structures in a dense hyaline stroma. Many of the tubules have two-layered epithelium. This is no proof of benignity. Because of these characteristics the tumor, however, was considered benign. But the patient died a few months later from generalized metastases. It was interesting to note that in the axillary metastases the same type of tubules with hyaline stroma was seen as in the primary tumor, in some places also with two cell layers.

The case was published by Gudjónsdóttir *et al.* (1971). Shortly after, several cases of the same type were published (Bhagavan et al., 1973). Nowadays even textbooks admit that florid mammillary adenomatosis can develop into carcinoma.

*Fig. 17-8*

*Mammillary adenocarcinoma.* Some details from the foregoing case. To the left we see tubules in hyaline stroma but to the right there are compact epithelial proliferations. Some but not all of the tubules have two-layered epithelium.

To the right, tubules at a higher magnification. The cells show a moderate atypia but we still have two-layered epithelium. In our opinion we cannot always base a diagnosis of benignity on these features only.

Florid mammillary adenomatosis is easily detected and therefore usually removed early. This may be why most cases behave in a benign way, but it is reasonable to suspect a potential malignancy and there is also reason to believe that there will be a progression from highly differentiated tumors to more aggressive forms, as exemplified by this case.

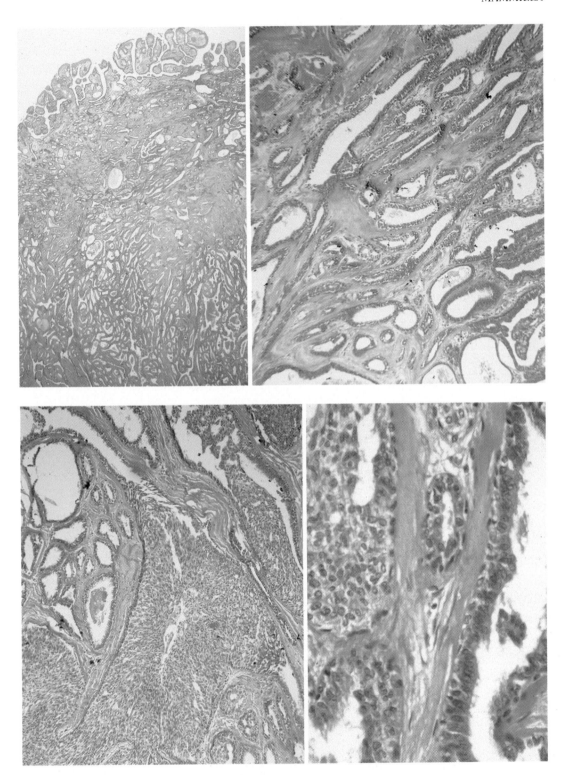

*Fig. 17-9*

*Lymphadenosis benigna cutis.* This disease has been illustrated because the mammilla is a typical location. It is especially seen in children or young people.

To the left, an overview with normal papillary epithelium on the surface. A dense infiltrate of lymphoid cells begins slightly beneath the epidermis. Light reaction centers are easily recognized. The narrow strip in the middle shows that the infiltrate of lymphocytes can be diffuse. To the right, typical reaction centers with a "starry sky" picture.

Lymphadenosis benigna cutis (Bäfverstedt's disease, Spiegler-Fendt's sarcoid) is a benign self-limiting disease that responds to small doses of radiation. In recent years it has been believed that most cases are preceded by insect bites but it is difficult to understand why the mammilla should be a predilection site for insect bites.

Lymphadenosis benigna cutis is an example of a disease which can be located anywhere in the skin but the mammilla is a predilection site.

*Fig. 17-10*

*Parasites (Demodex folliculorum).* To the left a small piece of the surface epithelium with a dilated hair follicle opening. Among the corny lamellae many, often curved, structures can be discerned.

To the right, at higher magnification, the organisms are more easily seen. They have a cuticle and the abdomen is grooved; at higher magnification one may even discern legs. Details can best be seen in direct smear preparations; less easily in paraffin embedded slides. The organisms are acarids with eight legs. These scavengers are normally present in the human skin and they eat bacteria etc. They are often seen in the mammilla which may have clumsy, dilated hair follicles.

These organisms, which cause no trouble, are ubiquitous in humans. The children will probably be infected very early through skin contact with their mothers. This can be easily accomplished during nursing.

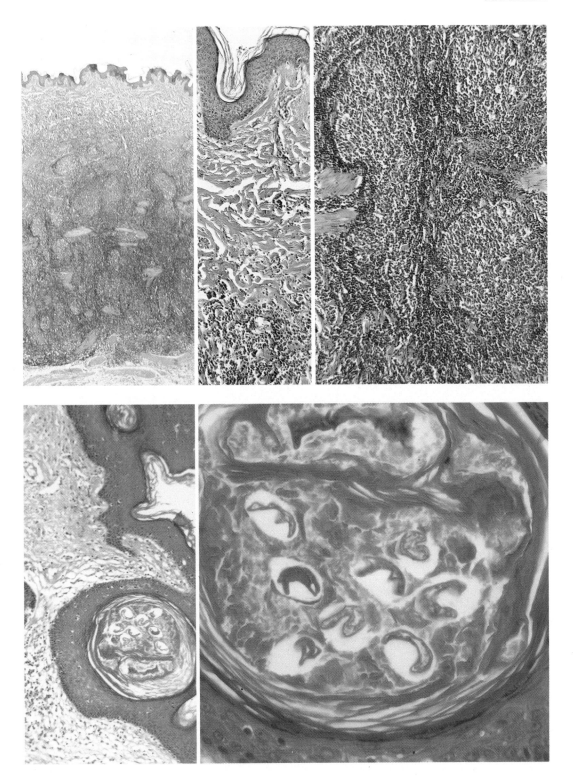

# Chapter 18

# Male Breast Diseases

*Fig. 18-1*

*Gynecomastia*. Development of breast tissue in the male is a very common finding. Many cases are spontaneous and idiopathic. Others are seen in cases with hormone producing tumors or liver lesions but most cases are iatrogenic.

Irrespective of the cause the appearance is mostly the same. The case here is rather characteristic. To the left, an overview. Gynecomastia is mostly of the juvenile type, i.e. reminiscent of the developing breast at menarche. This is characterized by proliferation of ducts but usually without lobules, as seen in the picture on the left. To the right, a higher magnification, showing ducts with slightly papillary epithelium. The ducts are often surrounded by a loose, myxomatous stroma not especially conspicuous in this case. Gynecomastia may show many histologic variations. Some cases (fat boys) consist mostly of fatty tissue with a few ducts. It is reasonable to assume that gynecomastia is caused by some hormonal disturbance, probably an imbalance in the sex hormone homeostasis. Many cases in young boys are unilateral. This could be explained by the fact that remnants of breast tissue may exist on only one side.

*Fig. 18-2*

*Gynecomastia with lobules*. It is often said that gynecomastia is characterized by development of ducts alone (juvenile type) but even development of lobules is not uncommon.

This is a case of a healthy 21-year-old man. To the left we see many ducts surrounded by connective tissue. In between there is plenty of fatty tissue. But we also see many ducts branching out in typical lobules. To the right, a higher magnification of a duct with several lobules (arrow).

Such lobule development is not uncommon in cases of carcinoma of the prostate treated with estrogens.

Breast carcinomas are also found in men (between 1:100 and 1:1000 in comparison with women). They are of the same types as carcinomas in women and will not be illustrated.

It has been claimed that lobular carcinoma does not exist in the male because there are no lobules (Scheike, 1974). We think this is simply a question of frequency because as we see in this case the prerequisite is there and in reality all types of carcinoma have been described in the male breast.

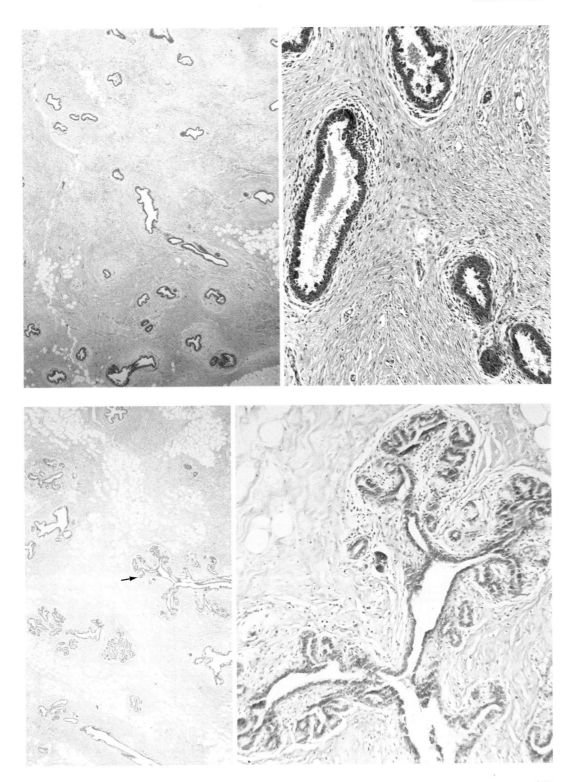

*Fig. 18-3*

*Gynecomastia after treatment with aldactone.* There are many causes of gynecomastia. Mostly it is estrogen induced, for example by estrogen producing tumors or liver diseases with defective destruction of estrogens. Most common is iatrogenic gynecomastia after estrogen treatment of carcinoma of the prostate. Very often gynecomastia is a complication of aldactone medication.

Epithelial proliferation is often vigorous and we have seen cases misdiagnosed as carcinoma at fine needle aspiration biopsy. The picture shows such a case. There is a cribriform and micropapillary pattern of the epithelial proliferation and there is also a slight atypia. We are not aware of any cases of male breast carcinoma after aldactone medication.

Aldactone also causes proliferative changes in the female breast (see Fig. 11-11). It is much more difficult to evaluate whether aldactone has carcinogenic properties in females.

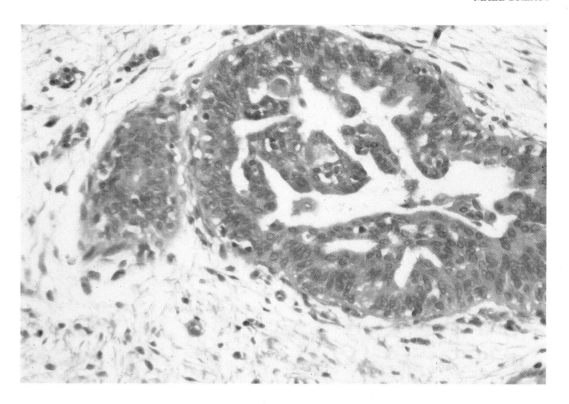

# Chapter 19

# Varia

*Fig. 19-1*

*Pleomorphic adenoma.* The breast glands are sweat gland derivatives. It seems natural then that sweat gland tumors also occur in the breasts, but it is highly disputable whether they really develop from breast tissue. These tumors may occur anywhere in the skin but when they happen to occur in the skin over the breast they are usually clinically interpreted as breast tissue tumors which may cause differential diagnostic problems.

The first case here is a type mostly seen in salivary glands, though it may appear anywhere in the skin, and is usually called chondroid syringoadenoma.

In this case it was a well palpable tumor rather close to the skin. At fine needle aspiration biopsy a diagnosis of mucinous carcinoma was made and an unnecessary mastectomy was done. Caution in diagnosis is warranted in such cases because these tumors are wholly benign.

The tumor is well demarcated and situated in the subcutaneous fatty tissue. The periphery shows epithelial strands in mucinous tissue but the eosinophil center is composed of chondro-osteoid tissue. See next figure.

*Fig. 19-2*

*Pleomorphic adenoma.* Details from the foregoing case. Left: In the upper part the well demarcated border without capsule. In the peripheral part there are epithelial strands with tubular structures. The strands are surrounded by a loose "myxomatous" tissue. In the lower part there is chondromatous tissue with calcifications and bone formation.

Right: A detail of the peripheral part, demonstrating the epithelial strands composed of rather regular cells. Some of the cells seem to "swim out" into the mucus, giving the impression of myxomatous tissue.

Pleomorphic adenomas are rare tumors of the breast and mostly located in the areolar region. They are usually small, up to 1 cm.

This type of tumor is rather common in dogs. There they often show rather vigorous proliferation but are said to behave in a benign fashion.

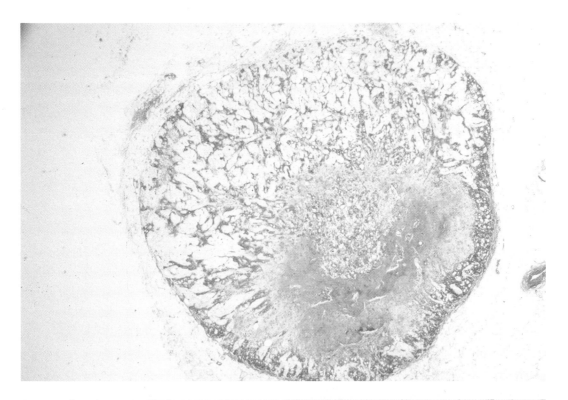

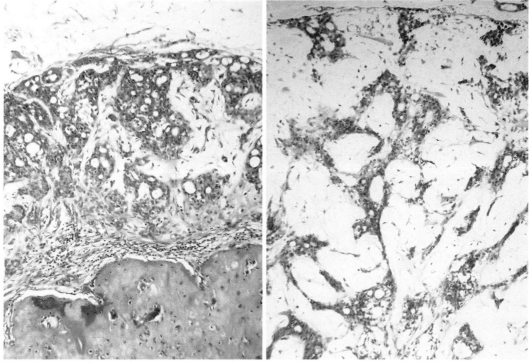

*Fig. 19-3*

*Eccrine spiradenoma*. The picture shows another example of sweat gland tumors rarely found in the breast skin. The tumors are often multiple and can be arranged like a chain of pearls. They are often tender, a typical feature. They are entirely benign.

To the left, two small, round tumors, very cellular and sharply delimited. To the right, the characteristic microscopic picture. The cells are arranged in small alveolar structures between very delicate stromal strands. There are two types of cell, one small and dark and one larger with light cytoplasm. Mitoses can be seen but they are few in number.

*Fig. 19-4*

*Myoepithelioma*. A 70-year-old woman has been operated upon 3 times during the last 15 years because of diffusely outlined lumps in one breast. The histologic picture has on the whole remained unchanged over the years.

To the left, a cellular part of the tumor. Tubular structures are layered "back to back". Some of the tubules have tall cylindrical epithelium but in many tubules there is an outer zone of clear cells, probably myothelial cells.

To the right, at higher magnification. The cells are not atypical but show some mitoses. Tumors of this type have been especially discussed by Hamperl.

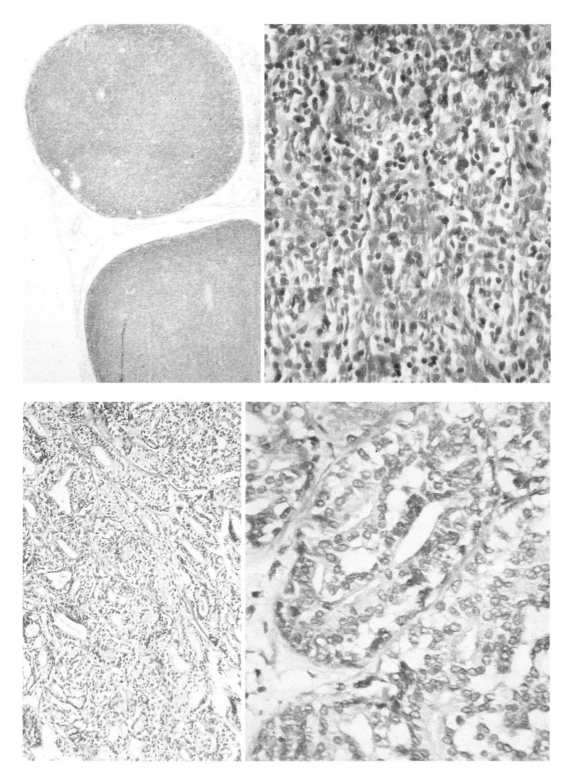

*Fig. 19-5*

*Myoepithelioma*. The same case. Left: The tubules are tortuous and narrowly layered.

To the right, at higher magnification one can see both the epithelium and the clear myothelial cells. It is curious to find that exactly the same type of tumor is illustrated in WHO's "Salivary gland tumours" as monomorphic clear cell adenoma.

It is conceivable that the same type of tumor exists both in salivary and mammary glands but they are *not* monomorphic. They are probably of a low grade of malignancy (compare the recurrences in this case).

*Fig. 19-6*

*Infiltrating fibromatosis*. These rare tumors can sometimes be palpated but mostly they are found incidentally at mammography. They are dense, stellate tumors and it is usually impossible to differentiate them from carcinoma. Fine needle aspiration may be of great value for diagnosis. They are often deeply located in connection with the deep fascia.

The picture shows a tumor with an uneven, spiky contour. The tumor consists of twisting bundles of fibromatous tissue. In the periphery there are often small round cell infiltrations (arrows).

These tumors are quite benign and seem to be of the same nature as other pseudotumors, such as nodular fasciitis or pseudosarcomas. They can be rather cellular and show many mitoses. It is only the problems of localization and the differential diagnosis from breast cancer that put them in a special position compared with nodular fasciitis in other localities (see next picture).

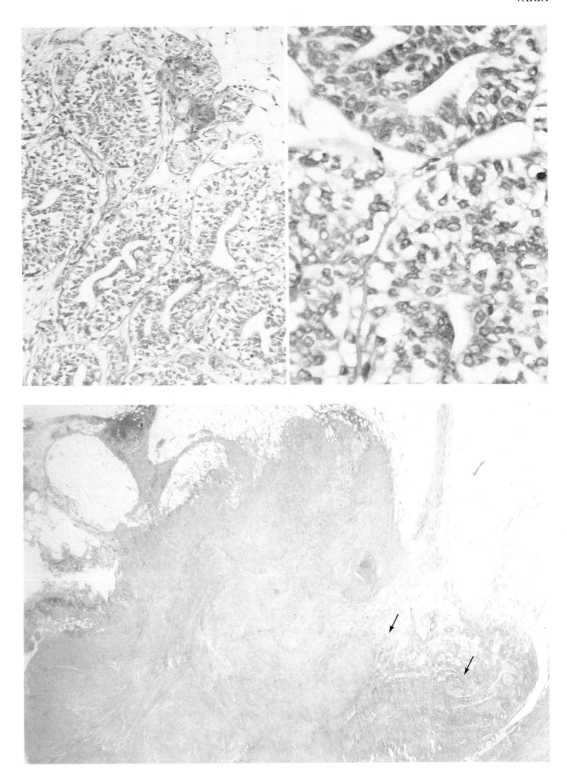

*Fig. 19-7*

*Infiltrating fibromatosis.* The picture shows details of the foregoing case.

To the left we see twisted bundles of fibroblasts among many thin-walled vessels, some with tiny round cell infiltrates. There is no cellular atypia.

To the right an elastin stained section. In the periphery there are some elastin fibers in a granulation tissue with several round cell infiltrates (arrows). Otherwise there is practically no elastin in these lesions (compare with radial scars).

Some cases of infiltrating fibromatosis appear to have a connection with trauma and earlier operative procedures. In other cases no etiologic incidents are evident.

It is imperative to bear these lesions in mind when viewing a carcinoma-like picture in the mammogram, and to require a positive carcinoma cytology before performing mastectomy.

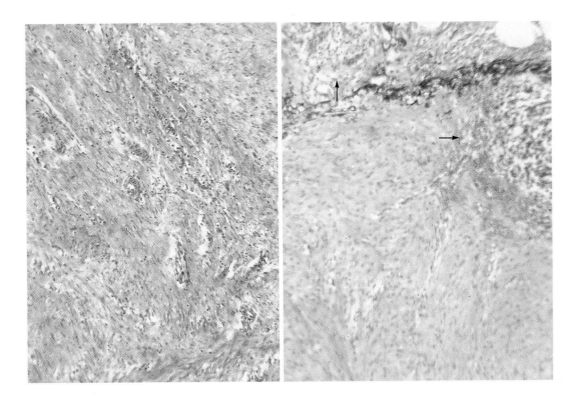

# Additional Reading

The literature about the breasts is immense and there can be no question of a complete list. The references are arranged under the different chapters, but there are some references appearing in several chapters. To save space they are listed here in the beginning.

There are three real goldmines of knowledge of breast diseases. We give them here alphabetically.

*Azzopardi, J.G.:* Problems in breast-pathology. Saunders, London, 1979.

*Bässler, R.:* Pathologie der Brustdrüse. Springer-Verlag, Berlin, 1978.

*Haagensen, C.D.:* Diseases of the breast. 2nd ed. Saunders, Philadelphia, 1971.

All these books contain a wealth of references and all of them contain many superb illustrations in black and white.

Special atlases are:

*McDivitt, R.W., Stewart, F.W. & Berg, J.W.:* Tumors of the breast. Atlas of tumor pathology. Armed Forces Institute of Pathology, Washington, D.C., 1968.

*Histological Typing of Breast Tumours.* World Health Organization, Geneva, 1981.

*Ahmed, A.:* Atlas of the ultrastructure of human breast diseases. Churchill Livingstone, Edinburgh, 1978.

Many illustrations of breast tumors are to be found in:

*Gowing, U.F.C.:* A colour atlas of tumour histopathology. Wolfe Medical Publications, London, 1980.

*Guthrie, W. & Fawkes, R.:* A colour atlas of surgical pathology. Wolfe Medical Publications, London, 1982.

Special problems in cancerogenesis are treated in the following atlas.

*Wellings, S.R., Jensen, H.M. & Marcum, R.G.:* Atlas of subgross pathology of the human breast with special reference to possible precancerous lesions. J. Natl. Cancer Inst. 1975, 55, 231-273.

In our atlas there are many references to an earlier monograph by us:

*Linell, F., Ljungberg, O. & Andersson, I.:* Breast carcinoma. Aspects of early stages, progression and related problems. Acta path. microbiol. scand. Sect. A. Suppl. 272, Munksgaard, Copenhagen, 1980.

Here many of the problems mentioned in the present atlas are more fully discussed.

Correlations between anatomic and mammographic pictures are to be found in the following atlases:

*Barth, V.:* Atlas of diseases of the breast. Synopsis of clinical, morphological, and radiological findings with a consideration of special investigation methods. G.Thieme Verlag, Stuttgart, 1979.

*Martin, J.E.:* Atlas of mammography. Histologic and mammographic correlations. Williams & Wilkins, Baltimore, 1982.

*Nathan, T.:* An atlas of normal and abnormal mammograms. Oxford, University Press, Oxford, 1982.

*Witt, H. & Bürger, H.:* Mammadiagnostik im Röntgenbild. Ein Atlas für die Praxis mit histologischen Schnitten. Walter de Gruyter, Berlin, 1981.

Our atlas does not deal with the important fine needle biopsy and therefore we refer to some comprehensive works on this theme:

*Kline, F.:* Aspiration biopsy cytology. Mosby Company, St. Louis, 1981.

*Koss, L.G.:* Diagnostic cytology and its histopathologic bases. Lippincott, Philadelphia, 1979.

*Schöndorf, H.:* Aspiration cytology of the

breast. Saunders, Philadelphia, 1978.

Zajicek, J.: Aspiration biopsy cytology. Part 1. Cytology of supradiaphragmatic organs. Karger, Basel, 1974.

In the following we list a sample of monographs and symposia that deal with different problems. Naturally many contributions in symposia have a rather ephemeral value but they often pose problems and give references. In this series there are books with little or no direct relevance for the pathologist but the latter must also have an interest in and knowledge of other aspects of breast lesions.

Andersson, I.: Mammographic screening for breast carcinoma. A cross-sectional randomized study of 45-69 year old women. Thesis, Malmö, 1980.

Angeli, A., Bradlow, H.L. & Dogliotti, L.: Endocrinology of cystic breast disease. Raven Press, New York, 1983.

Brennan, M.J., McGrath, C.M. & Rich, M.A.: Breast cancer. New concepts in etiology and control. Academic Press, New York, 1980.

Bulbrook, R.D. & Taylor, D.J.: Commentaries on research in breast disease. Vol. 1-2. Alan Liss Inc., New York, 1981.

Coombees, R.C., Powles, T.J., Ford, H.T. & Gazet, J.C.: Breast cancer management. Academic Press, London, 1981.

Cutler, M.: Tumors of the breast. Their pathology, symptoms, diagnosis and treatment. Lippincott, Philadelphia, 1962.

Donegan, W.L. & Spratt, J.S.: Cancer of the breast. Saunders, Philadelphia, 1979.

Feig, S.A. & McLelland, R.: Breast carcinoma. Current diagnosis and treatment. Masson, New York, 1983.

Frischbier, H.J.: Die Erkrankungen der weiblichen Brustdrüse. Georg Thieme Verlag, Stuttgart, 1982.

Gallager, H.St.: Early breast cancer. Detection and treatment. J.Wiley & Sons, New York, 1975.

Gallager, H.S., Leis, H.P.Jr., Snyderman, R.K. & Urban, J.A.: The breast. Mosby, St. Louis, 1978.

Grundmann, E. & Beck, L.: Early diagnosis of breast cancer. Gustav Fischer Verlag, Stuttgart, 1978.

Haagensen, C.D., Bodian, C. & Haagensen, D.E.: Breast carcinoma, risk and detection. Saunders, Philadelphia, 1981.

Hollmann, K.H., deBrux, J. & Verley, J.N.: New frontiers in mammary pathology. Plenum Press, New York, 1981.

Hoogstraten, B. & McDivitt, R.W.: Breast cancer. CRC Press, Boca Raton, 1981.

Hultborn, K.A. & Törnberg, B.: Mammary carcinoma. The biologic character of mammary carcinoma studied in 517 cases by a new form of malignancy grading. Acta Radiol., Suppl. 196, Stockholm, 1960.

Johnsén, C.: Breast disease. A clinical study with special reference to diagnostic procedures. Acta chir. scand. Suppl. 454, Stockholm, 1975.

Lundgren, B.: Single oblique view mammography. An efficient method for breast cancer screening. Thesis, Gävle, 1980.

Lynch, H.T.: Genetics and breast cancer. Van Nostrand, Reinhold Company, New York, 1981.

McGuire, W.L.: Breast cancer. Advances in research and treatment Vol. 1-4. Plenum Company, New York, 1977-1981.

Nohrman, B.: Cancer of the breast. A clinical study of 1042 cases treated at Radiumhemmet, 1934-1941. Acta radiol. Suppl. 77, Stockholm, 1949.

Rimsten, Å.: Diagnosis of breast tumours. With special reference to organization, clinical aspects and cytological procedures. Acta universitatis upsal., Uppsala, 1974.

Rutquist, L.E.: On breast cancer. Incidence and survival. Thesis, Stockholm, 1983.

Sandison, A.T.: An autopsy study of the adult

human breast: with special reference to pro-liferative epithelial changes of importance in the pathology of the breast. Natl. Cancer Inst., Monograph no. 8, 1962, 1-145.

Stoll, B.A.: New aspects of breast cancer. Heinemann, London, Vol. 1-5. 1977-1982.

Zinser, H.-K.: Mammakarzinom. Diagnose und Differentialdiagnose. Georg Thieme Verlag, Stuttgart, 1972.

The following references are listed according to the contents of the different chapters and alphabetically according to the name of the first author.

Naturally the bulk of references is concentrated on carcinoma. To facilitate the search of references we have tried to arrange them according to different types of carcinoma. However, we must leave many of the references to one heading: Carcinoma in general. We would like to emphasize that the selection of references is rather arbitrary because no one knows the literature so completely that an objectively justified choice is possible.

# References to Chapter 1. *The technique of study of breast specimens*

Fisher, B. & Slack, N.H.: Number of lymph nodes examined and the prognosis of breast carcinoma. Surg. Gynecol. Obstet. 1970, 131, 79-88.

Gibbs, N.M.: Large paraffin sections and chemical clearance of axillary tissues as a routine procedure in the pathological examination of the breast. Histopathology 1982, 6, 647-660.

Kay, S.: Evaluation of Rotter's lymph nodes in radical mastectomy specimens as a guide to prognosis. Cancer 1965, 18, 1441-1444.

Manton, S.L., Ferguson, D.J.P. & Andersson, T.J.: An automated technique for the rapid processing of breast tissue for subgross examination. J. clin. Pathol. 1981, 34, 1189-1191.

Wilkinson, E.J. & Hause, L.: Probability in lymph node sectioning. Cancer 1974, 33, 1269-1274.

# References to Chapters 2 and 11. *Normal anatomy*

Barwick, K., Kashgarian, M. & Rosen, P.P.: Clear-cell change within duct and lobular epithelium of the human breast. Pathol. Annu. 1982, 17, 319-328.

Davies, J.D.: Neural invasion in benign mammary dysplasia. J. Pathol. Bact. 1973, 109, 225-231.

Hamperl, H.: "Satellitengänge" in der Mamma bei proliferierender Mastopathie. Beitr. Pathol. 1972, 146, 339-350.

Hamperl, H.: Onkocyten und hyaline Einschlüsse in der menschlichen Mamma. Virch. Arch. Abt. B. 1972, 10, 88-92.

Hamperl, H.: Zellabschilferung in der Ausführungsgängen. Geburtsh. Frauenheilk. 1972, 32, 25-27.

Hamperl, H.: Epi-myotheliale Inseln. Virch. Arch. Abt. B. Cell. Pathol. 1974, 16, 89-93.

Hamperl, H.: Sekretionserscheinungen in der mastopathischen Brustdrüse. Virch. Arch. Abt. B. Cell. Path. 1975, 18, 73-81.

Kiaer, H.W. & Andersen, J.A.: Focal pregnancy-like changes in the breast. Acta path. microbiol. scand. 1977, 85, 931-941.

Kuzma, J.F.: Myoepithelial proliferations in the human breast. Amer. J. Pathol. 1943, 19, 473-489.

Leis, S.N., Palmer, B. & Östberg, G.: Gravid macromastia. Scand. J. Plast. Reconstr. Surg. 1974, 8, 247-249.

Theele, C. & Bässler, R.: Über Grössenordnung, Formen und Varianten der Drüsenläppchen der Mamma. Pathologe 1981, 2, 208-219.

Vogel, P.M., Georgiade, N.G., Fetter, B.F., Vogel, E.S. & McCarty, K.S.: The correlation of histologic changes in the human breast with the menstrual cycle. Am. J. Pathol. 1981, 104, 23-34.

Wolfe, J.N., Albert, S., Belle, S. & Salane, M.: Familial influences on breast parenchymal patterns. Cancer 1980, 46, 2433-2437.

## References to Chapters 3 and 12.
### Inflammatory changes

Ahmed, E.B., Ahmed, A., Rashid, A.T.M.F. & Wright, D.H.: Silicone lymphadenopathy: a report of two cases, one with concomitant malignant lymphoma. Histopathology 1982, 5, 133-141.

Andersson, I., Fex, G. & Pettersson, H.: Oil cyst of the breast following fat necrosis. Brit. J. Radiol. 1977, 50, 143-146.

Fletcher, A., Magrath, J.M., Riddell, R.H. & Talbot, I.C.: Granulomatous mastitis: a report of seven cases. J. clin. Pathol. 1982, 35, 941-945.

Gorton, G. & Linell, F.: Malignant tumours and sarcoid reactions in regional lymph nodes. Acta radiol. 1957, 47, 381-392.

Hamperl, H.: Herdförmige Epithelnekrose und Mikroverkalkung. Geburtsh. Frauenheilk. 1972, 32, 25-27.

Ingier, A.: Über obliterierende Mastitis. Virchows Arch. 1910, 198, 338-345.

Kessler, E. & Wolloch, Y.: Granulomatous mastitis: A lesion clinically simulating carcinoma. Am. J. Pathol. 1972, 58, 642-646.

Payne, R.L., Strauss, A.F. & Glasser, R.D.: Mastitis obliterans. Surgery. 1943, 141, 719-727.

Potter, B.T., Housley, E. & Thomson, D.: Giant-cell arteritis mimicking carcinoma of the breast. Brit. med. J. 1981, 282, 1665-1666.

Rickert, R.R., Rajan, S. & Newark, N.J.: Localized breast infarcts associated with pregnancy. Arch. Pathol. 1974, 97, 159-161.

Sandison, A.T. & Walker, J.C.: Inflammatory mastitis, mammary ductectasia, and mam-

millary fistula. Brit. J. Surg. 1962, 50, 57-64.

Wilhelms, J.L., Schrodt, G.R. & Makaffey, L.M.: Cholesterol granulomas of the breast. A lesion which clinically mimics carcinoma. Amer. J. clin. Pathol. 1982, 77, 592-597.

## References to Chapters 4 and 13.
### Benign tumors and tumor-like lesions

Albrecht, E.: Über Hamartome. Verh. Dtsch. ges. Pathol. 1906, 7, 153-157.

Arrigoni, M.G., Dockerty, M.B. & Judd, E.S.: The identification and treatment of mammary hamartoma. Surg. Gynecol. Obstet. 1971, 133, 577-582.

Buzanowski, F., Konakry, K., Harrison, E.G. & Payne, W.S.: Lobular carcinoma arising in fibroadenoma of the breast. Cancer 1975, 35, 450-456.

Carter, D.: Intraductal papillary tumours of the breast. A study of 78 cases. Cancer 1977, 39, 1689-1692.

Dyreborg, U. & Starklint, H.: Adenolipoma mammae. Acta radiol. 1975, 16, 362-366.

Eusebi, V. & Azzopardi, J.G.: Lobular endocrine neoplasia in fibroadenoma of the breast. Histopathology. 1980, 4, 413-428.

Fondo, E.Y., Rosen, P.P., Fracchia, A.A. & Urban, J.A.: The problem of carcinoma developing in a fibroadenoma. Recent experience at Memorial Hospital. Cancer 1979, 43, 563-567.

Goldman, R.L. & Friedman, N.B.: Carcinoma of the breast arising in fibroadenomas, with emphasis on lobular carcinoma. A clinicopathologic study. Cancer 1969, 23, 544-550.

Hendrick, J.W.: Intraductal papilloma of the breast. Surg. Gynecol. Obstet. 1957, 105, 215-222.

Hertel, B.F., Zaloudek, C. & Kempson, R.L.: Breast adenomas. Cancer 1976, 37, 2891-2905.

Hessler, C., Schnyder, P. & Ozello, L.: Hamartoma of the breast. Diagnostic observations of 16 cases. Radiology 1978, 126, 95-98.

*Hogeman, K.E. & Östberg, G.:* Three cases of postlactational breast tumor of a peculiar type. Acta pathol. microbiol. scand. 1968, 73, 169-176.

*Kiaer, H.W., Kiaer, W.W., Linell, F. & Jacobson, S.:* Extreme duct papillomatosis of the juvenile breast. Acta pathol. microbiol. scand. Sect. A. 1979, 87, 353-359.

*Kronsbein, H. & Bässler, R.:* Pathomorphologie und Diagnostik sogenannter Hamartoma der Mamma. Der Pathologe 1982, 3, 310-318.

*Linell, F., Östberg, G., Söderström, J., Andersson, I., Hildell, J. & Ljungquist, U.:* Breast hamartomas. An important entity in mammary pathology. Virch. Arch. A. 1979, 383, 253-264.

*Ljungquist, U., Andersson, I., Hildell, J. & Linell, F.:* Mammary hamartoma. A benign breast lesion. Acta chir. scand. 1979, 145, 227-230.

*Moross, T., Lang, A.P. & Mahoney, L.:* Tubular adenoma of breast. Arch. Pathol. lab. Med. 1983, 107, 84-86.

*Murad, T.M., Swaid, S. & Pritchett, P.:* Malignant and benign papillary lesions of the breast. Hum. Pathol. 1977, 8, 379-390.

*Prym, P.:* Pseudoadenome, Adenome und Mastome der weiblichen Brustdrüse. Beitr. Pathol. Anat. 1928, 81, 1-44, 221-263.

*Rosen, P.P., Cantrell, B., Mullen, D.L. & dePalo, A.:* Juvenile papillomatosis (Swiss cheese disease) of the breast. Progress in Surg. Pathol. I, Masson, New York, 1980.

*Sigfusson, B.F., Andersson, I. & Ljungberg, O.:* Percutaneous injection of contrast medium into breast lesions for radiographic exclusion of malignancy. Brit. J. Radiol. 1982, 55, 26-31.

*Spalding, J.E.:* Adenolipoma and lipoma of the breast. Guy's Hosp. Rep. 1945, 94, 80-89.

# References to Chapters 5 and 14.
## Cystic breast disease and related conditions

*Ahmed, A.:* The myoepithelium in cystic hyperplastic mastopathy. J. Pathol. 1974, 113, 209-215.

*Ashikari, R., Huvos, A.G., Snyder, R.E., Lucas, J.C., Hutter, R.V.P., McDivitt, R.W. & Schottenfeld, D.:* A clinicopathologic study of atypical lesions of the breast. Cancer 1974, 33, 310-317.

*Azzopardi, J.G. & Laurini, R.N.:* Elastosis in breast cancer. Cancer 1974, 33, 174-183.

*Bahrmann, E.:* Die Mastopathie als Vorläufer des Mammakarzinoms. Dtsch. Gesund. Wes. 1962, 17, 1762-1765.

*Berning, H. & Bücker, J.:* Mastopathia cystica (apokrine Drüsencysten) und Carcinom. Virch. Arch. 1937, 298, 728-742.

*Böhmig, R.:* Die Epithelproliferationen bei der Mastopathia fibrosa cystica. Zbl. allg. Pathol. pathol. Anat. 1952, 89, 297-313.

*Böhmig, R.:* Die Bildungsarten, Entwicklungsstadien und Wachstumsstufen des Carcinoms am Beispiel der Epithelproliferationen der Brustdrüse. Z. Krebsforsch. 1953, 59, 11-27.

*Böhmig, R.:* Mastopathia fibrosa cystica, ihre Epithelproliferationen und deren Beziehungen zum Carcinom. Erg. allg. Pathol. Pathol. Anat. 1964, 45, 39-116.

*Clement, P.B. & Azzopardi, J.G.:* Microglandular adenosis of the breast – a lesion simulating tubular carcinoma. Histopathol. 1983, 7, 169-180.

*Contesso, G., Rouëssé, J. & Jacquemier, J.:* Histologie des lésions précancéreuses du sein. J. Gynaecol Obst. Biol. Repr. 1975, 4, 5-20.

*Davies, J.D.:* Neural invasion in benign mammary dysplasia. J. Pathol. 1973, 109, 225-231.

*Davies, J.D.:* Hyperelastosis, obliteration and fibrous plaques in major ducts of the human breast. J. Pathol. 1973, 110, 13-26.

*Dawson, E.K.:* Fibrosing adenosis. Edinburgh med. J. 1954, 61, 391-491.

*Dawson, E.K.:* "Precancerous conditions" of the breast. Brit. J. Radiol. 1948, 21, 590-594.

*Donnelly, P.K., Baker, K.W., Carney, J.A. & O'Fallon, W.M.:* Benign breast lesions and subsequent breast carcinoma in Rochester, Minnesota. Mayo Clin. Proc. 1975, 50, 650-656.

*Egger, H., Weishaar, J. & ·Hamperl, H.:* "Sterne" im Mammogramm-Karzinome und "strahlige Narben". Geburtsh. Frauenheilk. 1976, 36, 547-553.

*Egger, H. & Dressler, W.:* A contribution to the natural history of breast cancer. I. Duct obliteration with periductal elastosis in the centre of breast cancers. Arch. Gynecol. 1982, 231, 191-198.

*Eusebi, V. & Azzopardi, J.G.:* Vascular infiltration in benign breast disease. J. Pathol. 1976, 18, 9-25.

*Ewing, J.:* Neoplastic diseases. Saunders, Philadelphia, 1940, 541-542.

*Fenoglio, C. & Lattes, R.:* Sclerosing papillary proliferations in the female breast. A benign lesion often mistaken for carcinoma. Cancer 1974, 33, 691-700.

*Fisher, E.R., Palekar, A.S., Kotwal, N. & Lipana, N.:* A nonencapsulated sclerosing lesion of the breast. Amer. J. clin. Pathol. 1979, 71, 240-246.

*Foote, F.W. & Stewart, F.W.:* Comparative studies of cancerous versus non-cancerous breasts. Ann. Surg. 1945, 121, 6-53, 197-222.

*Goldenberg, V.E., Goldenberg, N.S. & Sommers, S.C.:* Comparative ultrastructure of atypical ductal hyperplasia, intraductal carcinoma and infiltrating ductal carcinoma of the breast. Cancer 1969, 24, 1152-1169.

*Gould, V.E., Rogers, D.R. & Sommers, S.C.:* Epithelial-nerve intermingling in benign breast lesions. Arch. Pathol. 1975, 99, 596-598.

*Grove, J.S., Goodman, M.J., Gilbert, F. & Clyde, D.:* Factors associated with breast structure in breast cancer patients. Cancer 1979, 43, 1895-1899.

*Hamperl, H.:* Epithelzotten und Epithelnetze. Virch. Arch. Abt. B. Zellpatol. 1973, 12, 104-111.

*Hamperl, H.:* Strahlige Narben und obliterierende Mastopathie. Virch. Arch. A. Path. Anat. Histol. 1975, 369, 55-68.

*Hutter, R.V.P.:* The pathologists role in minimal breast cancer. Cancer 1971, 28, 1527-1536.

*Kern, W.H. & Brooks, R.N.:* Atypical epithelial hyperplasia associated with breast cancer and fibrocystic disease. Cancer 1969, 24, 668-675.

*Kiaer. W.:* Relation of fibroadenomatosis ("chronic mastitis") to cancer of the breast. Munksgaard, Copenhagen, 1954.

*Kiaer, W.:* The problem of "chronic mastitis" with epitheliosis. J. clin. Pathol. 1969, 23, 92.

*Kodlin, D., Winger, E.E., Morgenstern, N.L. & Chen, U.:* Chronic mastopathy and breast cancer. A follow up study. Cancer 1977, 39, 2603-2607.

*Krückemeyer, K.:* Dysplasien des Brustdrüsenepithel und ihre Beziehungen zum Mamma-Karzinom. Zbl. Gynäkol. 1969, 91, 993-1001.

*Liedberg, N.:* Über Mastopathia cystica. Acta chir. scand. 1931, 68, 369-424.

*Lindgren, S.:* On mastopathia cystica. Its frequency at post mortem examination and the possibility of its spontaneous regression. Acta chir. scand. 1937, 79, 119-140.

*Love, S.M., Gelman, R.S. & Silen, W.:* Fibrocystic "disease" of the breast – a nondisease? N. Engl. med. J. 1982, 307, 1010-1014.

*Lundmark, C.:* Breast cancer and elastosis. Cancer 1972, 30, 1195-1201.

Macgillivray, J.B. The problem of "chronic mastitis" with epitheliosis. J. clin. Pathol. 1969, 22, 340-347.

Martinez-Hernandez, A., Francis, D.J. & Silverberg, St.G.: Elastosis and other stromal reactions in benign and malignant breast tissue. An ultrastructural study. Cancer 1977, 40, 700-706.

Meyer, E.C. & Liebow, A.: Relationship of interstitial pneumonia, honey-combing and atypical epithelial proliferation to cancer of the lung. Cancer 1965, 18, 322-351.

Muir, R.: The evolution of the carcinoma of the mamma. J. Pathol. Bact. 1941, 52, 155-172.

Nizze, H.: Fibrous cystic mastopathy and epitheliosis in the opposite breast of mammary carcinoma patients. Oncology 1973, 28, 319-330.

Petri, M.: Neoplastic tissue: The so-called cancer bell. Dan. med. Bull. 1979, 26.

Rickert, R.R., Kalisher, L. & Hutter, R.V.P.: Indurative mastopathy: A benign sclerosing lesion of breast with elastosis which may simulate carcinoma. Cancer 1981, 47, 561-571.

Roessle, R.: Die Narbenkrebse der Lungen. Schweiz. med. Wschr. 1943, 73, 1200-1203.

Riedel, G.: Die Entwicklung und Entartung der elastischen Gewebes in der senilen Mamma. Virch. Arch. 1925, 256, 243-267.

Robertson, A.J., Brown, R.A., Cree, I.A., MacGillivray, J.B., Slidders, W. & Swanson, B.J.: Prognostic value of measurement of elastosis in breast carcinoma. J. clin. Pathol. 1981, 34, 738-743.

Rosen, P.P.: Microglandular adenosis. Anatomic pathology. Amer. Society Clin. Pathologists, Chicago, 1978.

Rosen, P.P.: Microglandular adenosis. A benign lesion simulating invasive mammary carcinoma. Amer. J. Surg. Pathol. 1983, 7, 137-144.

Sandison, A.T.: A study of surgically removed specimens of breast, with special reference to sclerosing adenosis. J. clin. Pathol. 1958, 11, 101-109.

Scheel, O.: Über Neubildung des elastischen Gewebes in Karzinomen, besonders der Mamma. Beitr. pathol. Anat. 1908, 187-198.

Semb, C.: Pathologico-anatomical and clinical investigations of fibroadenomatosis cystica mammae and its relation to other pathological conditions in the mammae, especially cancer. Acta chir. scand. 1928, Suppl. 10, 1-428.

Sigfusson, B.F., Andersson, I., Aspegren, K., Janzon, L., Linell, F. & Ljungberg, O.: Clustered breast calcifications. Acta Radiol. 1983, 24, 273-281.

Stegner, H.E.: Morphologie prämaligner und maligner Veränderungen der Mamma. Gynäkologe 1977, 10, 129-139.

Taylor, H.B. & Norris, H.J.: Epithelial invasion of nerves in benign diseases of the breast. Cancer 1967, 20, 2245-2249.

Toker, C.: Small cell dysplasia and in situ carcinoma of the mammary ducts and lobules. J.Pathol. 1974, 164, 47-52.

Torhorst, J.: Prognostische Bedeutung von pathologisch-anatomischen Befunden bei Mastopathie und Mamma-karzinom, Ther. Umschau 1976, 33, 781-785.

Tremblay, G., Buell, R.H. & Seemayer, Th.A.: Elastosis in benign sclerosing ductal proliferation of the female breast. Amer. J. Surg. Pathol. 1977, 1, 155-159.

Urban, J.A. & Adair, F.E.: Sclerosing adenosis. Cancer 1949, 2, 625-634.

Wellings, S.R. & Jensen, H.M: On the origin and progression of ductal carcinoma in the breast. J. Natl. Cancer Inst. 1973, 50, 1111-1118.

# References to Chapters 6 and 15.
*Carcinomas*

## Carcinoma in general

*Ackerman, L.V.:* Carcinoma of the breast. Pathologic changes correlated with diagnosis, treatment and prognosis. J. Ind. State Med. Ass. 1952, 45, 891-899.

*Ackerman, L.V. & Katzenstein, A.L.:* The concept of minimal breast cancer and the pathologist's role in the diagnosis of "early carcinoma". Cancer 1977, 39, 2755-2763.

*Adami, H.-O., Hansen, J., Jung, B. & Rimsten, Å.:* Characteristics of familial breast cancer in Sweden: Absence of relation to age and unilateral versus bilateral disease. Cancer 1981, 48, 1688-1695.

*Ahmed, A.:* The myoepithelium in human breast carcinoma. J.Pathol. 1974, 113, 129-135.

*Ahmed, A.:* Calcification in human breast carcinomas: ultrastructural observations. J. Pathol. 1975, 117, 247-251.

*Andersson, I., Andrén, L., Hildell, J., Linell, F., Ljungquist, U. & Pettersson, H.:* Breast cancer screening with mammography. A population-based, randomized trial with mammography as the only screening mode. Radiology 1979, 132, 273-276.

*Ashikari, R., Huvos, A.G. & Snyder, R.E.:* Prospective study of non-infiltrating carcinoma of the breast. Cancer 1977, 39, 435-439.

*Bahrmann, E.:* Über eine gelbartige dunkle Verfärbung des Fettgewebes im Bereiche von Carcinomen, besonders der Mamma. Langenbachs Arch. klin. Chir. 1954, 279, 109-111.

*Berge, T. & Lundberg, S.:* Cancer in Malmö 1958-1969. An autopsy study. Acta pathol. microbiol. scand. Sect. A., 1977, Suppl. 260, Munksgaard, Copenhagen.

*Bloom, H.J.G. & Richardson, W.W.:* Histological grading and prognosis in breast cancer. A study of 1409 cases of which 359 have been followed for 15 years. Brit. J. Cancer 1957, 11, 359-377.

*Bloom, H.J.G., Richardson, W.W. & Harries,E.J.:* Natural history of untreated breast cancer (1805-1933). Comparison of untreated and treated cases according to histological grade of malignancy. Brit. Med. J. 1962, 2, 213-221.

*van Bogaert,L.J. & Hermans, J.:* Importance of spicules on clinical staging of carcinoma of the breast. Surg. Gyn. Obst. 1977, 144, 356-358.

*van Bogaert, L.-J.:* Histologic typing of breast cancer. Letter to Editor. Acta pathol. microbiol. scand. Sect. A. 1980, 88A, 415-416; Reply by Linell, F., Ljungberg, O. & Andersson, I.: 1980, 88A, 416.

*van Bogaert, L.J. & Maldague, P.:* Histologic classification of pure primary epithelial breast cancer. Hum. Pathol. 1978, 9, 175-180.

*Borgström, S. & Linell, F.:* In preparation.

*Broberg, A., Glas, U., Gustafsson, S.A., Hellström, L. & Somell, A.:* Relationship between mammographic pattern and estrogen receptor content in breast cancer. Breast Cancer Res. Treatment 1983, 3, 201-207.

*Brownstein, M.H., Wolf, M. & Bikowski, J.B.:* Cowden's disease. A cutaneous marker of breast cancer. Cancer 1978, 41, 2393-2398.

*Carter, D. & Smith, R.R.L.:* Carcinoma in situ of the breast. Cancer 1977, 40, 1189-1193.

*Chabon, A.B., Goldberg, J.D. & Veust, L.:* Carcinoma of the breast: Interrelationships among histopathologic features, estrogen receptor activity, and age of the patient. Hum. Pathol. 1982, 14, 368-372.

*Clark, W.H., Folberg, R. & Ainsworth, A.M.:* Tumor progression in primary human cutaneous malignant melanomas. In Human malignant melanoma, edited by Clark, Goldman & Mastrangelo. Grune & Stratton, New York, 1979.

*Delides, G.S., Garas, G., Gergonli, G., Jiortziotis, D., Lena, J., Liva, Th. & Elemenoglou, J.:* Intralaboratory variations in the grading of breast carcinoma. Arch. Pathol. lab. Med. 1982, 106, 126-128.

*Ewing, J.:* Classification of mammary cancer. Ann. Surg. 1935, 102, 249-252.

*Feldman, J.G., Carter, A.C., Nicastic, A.D. & Hosat, S.T.:* Breast self-examination, relationship to stage of breast cancer at diagnosis. Cancer 1981, 47, 2740-2745.

*Fisher, E.R., Gregorio, R.M. & Fisher, B.:* The pathology of invasive cancer. Cancer 1975, 36, 1-84.

*Fisher, E.R., Palekar, A.S., Sass, R. & Fisher, B.:* Scar cancers: pathologic findings from the National Surgical Adjuvant Breast Project (Protocol no. 4). IX. Breast Cancer Res. Treatment, 1983, 3, 39-59.

*Fisher, E.R., Swamidoss, S., Lee, C.H., Rockette, H., Redmond, C. & Fisher, B.:* Detection and significance of occult axillary node metastases in patients with invasive breast cancer. Cancer 1978, 42, 2025-2031.

*Fisher, E.R., Palekar, A., Rockette, H., Redmond, C. & Fisher, B.:* Significance of axillary nodal micro- and macrometastases. Cancer 1978, 42, 2032-2038.

*Foot, N.C.:* A simpler classification of mammary tumors. Arch. Pathol. 1942, 33, 905-916.

*Foote, F.W. & Stewart, F.W.:* Comparative studies of cancerous versus noncancerous breasts. Ann. Surg. 1945, 121, 6-53, 197-222.

*Foote, F.W. & Stewart, F.W.:* A histologic classification of carcinoma of the breast. Surgery 1946, 19, 74-99.

*Foulds, L.:* Neoplastic development, Vols. 1 and 2. Academic Press, London, 1969 and 1975.

*Fracchia, A.A., Rosen, P.P. & Ashikari, R.:* Primary carcinoma of the breast without axillary lymph node metastases. Surg. Gynecol. Obstet. 1980, 151, 375-378.

*Freedman, L.S., Edwards, D.N., McConnell, E.M. & Downham, D.Y.:* Histological grade and other prognostic factors in relation to survival of patients with breast cancer. Brit. J. Cancer 1979, 40, 44-55.

*Gallager, H.S. & Martin, J.E.:* An orientation to the concept of minimal breast cancer. Cancer 1971, 28, 1505-1507.

*Gallager, H.S. & Martin, J.E.:* Early phases in the development of breast cancer. Cancer 1969, 24, 1170-1178.

*Gert, J., Hebert, H., Gentile, A., Laval, C. & Guerin, P.:* Cancer du sein. Encyclopédie Médico-chirurgicale 1975, 865 $A^{10} - F^{10}$, 1977, 870 $A^{10} - A^{20}$, 1980, 871 $A^{10} - A^{40}$.

*Hagemeister, F.B., Buzdar, A.N., Luna, M.A. & Blumenschein, G.R.:* Causes of death in breast cancer. A clinico-pathologic study. Cancer 1980, 46, 162-167.

*Heuser, L., Spratt, J.S. & Polk, H.C., Jr.:* Growth rates of primary breast cancers. Cancer 1979, 43, 1888-1894.

*Hutter, R.P.V.:* The pathologist's role in minimal breast cancer. Cancer 1971, 28, 1527-1536.

*Kern, W.H. & Mikkelsen, W.P.:* Small carcinomas of the breast. Cancer 1971, 28, 948-954.

*Linell, F. & Ljungberg, O.:* Breast carcinoma. Progressing of tubular carcinoma and a new classification. Acta pathol. microbiol. scand. Sect. A. 1980, 88, 59-60.

*Linell, F., Ljungberg, O. & Andersson, I.:* Breast carcinoma. Aspects of early stages, progression and related problems. Acta pathol. microbiol. scand. Sect. A. Suppl. 272, Munksgaard, 1980.

*Linell, F., Ljungberg, O. & Andersson, I.:* Brustkarzinom. Frühstadien, Progression und verwandte Probleme. Pathologe 1981, 2,

150-155.

Lynch, H.T., Fain, P.M., Golgar, D., Albano, W.A., Maillard, J.A. & McKenna, P.: Familial breast cancer and its recognition in an oncologic clinic. Cancer 1981, 47, 2730-2739.

Miller, A.B.: Screening for breast cancer. Breast Cancer Res. Treatment 1983, 3, 143-156.

Mombo, N.C. & Gallager, H.S.: Carcinoma of the breast. The prognostic significance of extranodal extension of axillary disease. Cancer 1977, 39, 2280-2285.

Muir, R.: The evolution of carcinoma of the mamma. J. Pathol. Bact. 1941, 52, 155-172.

Möbius, G. & Wittstock, G.: Zum biologischen Verhalten des Mammacarcinoms in Abhängigkeit vom histologischen Typ. Frankf. Z. Pathol. 1965, 74, 659-669.

Ozello, L. & Saupitak, P.: Epithelial-stromal junction of intraductal carcinoma of the breast. Cancer 1970, 26, 1186-1198.

Ozello, L.: Ultrastructure of intra-epithelial carcinomas of the breast. Cancer 1971, 28, 1508-1515.

Pontén, J., Bengtsson, A., Killander, D., Bondeson, L., Linell, F. & Ljungberg, O.: In preparation.

Rosen, P.P.: The pathological classification of human mammary carcinoma: Past, present and future. Ann. clin. lab. Sci. 1979, 9, 144-156.

Rosen, P.P.: Axillary lymph node metastases in patients with occult non-invasive breast carcinoma. Cancer 1980, 46, 1298-1306.

Saphir, O.: A text on systemic pathology. Grune & Stratton, New York, 1958.

Shah, J.P., Rosen, P.P. & Robbins, G.F.: Pitfalls of local excision in the treatment of carcinoma of the breast. Surg. Gynecol. Obst. 1973, 136, 721-725.

Sharkey, F.E.: Biological meaning of stage and grade in human breast cancer: review and hypothesis. Breast Cancer Res. a. Treatment 1982, 2, 299-322.

Schiödt, T.: Breast carcinoma. A histologic and prognostic study of 650 follow-up cases. Munksgaard, Copenhagen, 1966.

Sigfusson, B. & Andersson, I.: In preparation.

Sommers, S.C.: Histologic changes in incipient carcinoma of the breast. Cancer 1969, 23, 822-825.

Stegner, H.E.: Die Rolle des Pathologen in der stadiengerechten Therapie des Mamma-karzinoms. Pathologe 1982, 3, 137-148.

Stenkvist, B., Bengtsson, E., Eriksson, O., Jarkrans, T., Nordin, S. & Westman-Naeser, S.: Histopathological systems of breast cancer classification: reproducibility and clinical significance. J. clin. Pathol. 1983, 36, 392-398.

Tulusan, A.H., Grünsteidel, W., Ramming, I. & Egger, H.: A contribution to the natural history of breast cancer. III. Changes in the basement membranes in breast cancers with stromal microinvasion. Arch. Gynecol. 1982, 231, 209-218.

Wanebo, H.J., Huvos, A.G. & Urban, J.A.: Treatment of minimal breast cancer. Cancer 1974, 33, 349-357.

Wellings, S.R. & Jensen, H.M.: On the origin and progression of ductal carcinoma in the breast. J. Natl. Cancer Inst. 1973, 50, 1111-1118.

# Tubular and tubuloductal carcinoma

Andersson, I., Andrén, L., Hildell, J., Linell, F., Ljungquist, U. & Pettersson, H.: Breast cancer screening with mammography. A population-based, randomized trial with mammography as the only screening mode. Radiology 1979, 132, 273-276.

van Bogaert, L.J.: Clinicopathologic hallmarks of mammary tubular carcinoma. Hum. Pathol. 1982, 13, 558-562.

Carstens, P.H.B., Huvos, A.G., Foote, F.W. & Ashikari, R.: Tubular carcinoma of the breast: a clinico-pathologic study of 35 cases. Amer. J. clin. Pathol. 1972, 58, 231-238.

Carstens, P.H.B.: Tubular carcinoma of the breast. A study of frequency. Amer. J. clin. Pathol. 1978, 70, 204-210.

Caspersson, T. & Santesson, L.: Studies on protein-metabolism in the cells of epithelial tumors. Acta Radiol. Suppl. 46, Stockholm, 1942.

Cooper, H.S., Patchefsky, A.S. & Krall, R.A.: Tubular carcinoma of the breast. Cancer 1978, 42, 2334-2342.

Deos, Ph.D. & Norris, H.J.: Well-differentiated (tubular) carcinoma of the breast. A clinicopathologic study of 145 pure and mixed cases. Amer. J. clin. Pathol. 1982, 78, 1-7.

Egger, H., Tulusan, A.H. & Schneider, M.L.: A contribution to the natural history of breast cancer. II. Precursors and lesions associated with small cancers of the breast. Arch. Gynecol. 1982, 231, 199-308.

Erlandson, R.A. & Carstens, P.H.B.: Ultrastructure of tubular carcinoma of the breast. Cancer 1972, 29, 987-995.

Eusebi, V., Betts, C.M. & Bussolati, G.: Tubular carcinoma: a variant of secretory breast carcinoma. Histopathology 1979, 3, 407-419.

Feig, S.A., Shaber, G.S., Patchefsky, A.S., Schwartz, G.F., Eideken, J. & Nerlinger, R.E.: Tubular carcinoma of the breast. Mammographic appearance and pathological correlation. Radiology 1978, 129, 311-314.

Fisher, E.R., Palekar, A.S., Sass, R. & Fisher, B.: Scar cancers: pathologic findings from the National Surgical Adjuvant Breast Project (Protocol no. 4). IX. Breast Cancer Res. Treatment 1983, 3, 39-59.

Fisher, E.R., Gregorio, R.M., Redmond, C. & Fisher, B.: Tubulolobular invasive breast carcinoma: a variant of lobular invasive cancer. Hum. Pathol. 1977, 8, 679-683.

Hamperl, H.: Zur Frage des Carcinoma tubulare der Mamma und der Einteilung der Mammacarcinoma des Menschen. Z. Krebsforsch. 1974, 81, 181-191.

Lagios, M.D., Rose, M.R. & Margolin, F.R.: Tubular carcinoma of the breast. Association with multicentricity, bilaterality, and family history of mammary carcinoma. Amer. J. clin. Pathol. 1980, 73, 25-30.

McDivitt, R.W., Boyce, W. & Garsell, D.: Tubular carcinoma of the breast. Clinical and pathological observations concerning 135 cases. Amer. J. Surg. Pathol. 1982, 6, 401-411.

Oberman, H.A. & Fidler, W. J.: Tubular carcinoma of the breast. Amer. J. Surg. Pathol. 1979, 3, 387-395.

Page, D.L., Dixon, J.M., Anderson, F.J., Lee, D. & Stewart, H.J.: Invasive cribriform carcinoma of the breast. Histopathology 1983, 7, 525-536.

Patchefsky, A.S., Schaber, G.S., Schwartz, G.F., Feig, S.A. & Nerlinger, R.E.: The pathology of breast cancer detected by mass population screening. Cancer 1977, 40, 1659-1670.

Peters, G.N., Wolff, M. & Haagensen, C.D.: Tubular carcinoma of the breast. Clinical pathologic correlations based on 100 cases. Ann. Surg. 1981, 193, 138-149.

Taylor, H.B. & Norris, H.J.: Well-differentiated carcinoma of the breast. Cancer 1970, 25, 687-692.

Tobon, H. & Salazar, H.: Tubular caricnoma of the breast. Clinical, histological and ultrastructural observations. Arch. Pathol. lab. Med. 1977, 101, 310-316.

Tremblay, G.: Elastosis in tubular carcinoma of the breast. Arch. Pathol. 1974, 98, 302-307.

Wellington, J., Recant, W. & Swerdlow, M.A.: Comparative ultrastructure of tubular carcinoma and sclerosing adenosis of the breast. Cancer 1976, 38, 180-186.

## Comedo carcinoma

*Ashikari, R., Hajdu, S.J. & Robbins, G.F.:* Intraductal carcinoma of the breast (1960-1969). Cancer 1971, 28, 1182-1187.

*Bloodgood, J.C.:* Comedo carcinoma (or comedo-adenoma) of the female breast. Ann. J. Cancer 1934, 22, 842-853.

*Carter, D., Orr, S.L. & Merino, M.J.:* Intracystic papillary carcinoma of the breast. After mastectomy, radiotherapy or excisional biopsy alone. Cancer 1983, 52, 14-19.

*Contesso, G. & Petit, J.E.:* Les adenocarcinomas intracanalaires non infiltrants du sein. Bull. Cancer 1979, 66, 1-8.

*Cowen, P.N.:* Recognition of intraduct mammary carcinoma. Letter to the Editor. J. clin Pathol. 1980, 33, 797.

*Fisher, E.R., Palekar, A.S., Redmond, C., Barton, B. & Fisher, B.:* Invasive papillary cancer. Amer. J. clin. Pathol. 1980, 73, 313-322.

*Hamperl, H.:* Das sogenannte Schweissdrüsen-carcinom der Mamma. Eine Übersicht. Z. Krebsforsch. 1977, 88, 105-109.

*Lagios, M.D., Westdahl, Ph.R., Margolin, F.R. & Rose, M.E.R.:* Duct carcinoma in situ. Relationship of extent of noninvasive disease to the frequency of occult invasion, multicentricity, lymph node metastases, and short-term treatment failures. Cancer 1982, 50, 1309-1314.

*McDivitt, R.W., Holleb, A.J. & Foote, F.W.Jr.:* Prior breast disease in patients treated for papillary carcinoma. Arch. Pathol. 1968, 85, 117-124.

*Millis, R.R. & Thynne, G.S.J.:* In situ intraduct carcinoma of the breast: a long term follow-up study. Brit. J. Surg. 1975, 62, 957-962.

*Moore, O.S. & Foote, F.W., Jr.:* The relatively favorable prognosis of medullary carcinoma of the breast. Cancer 1949, 2, 635-642.

*Mossler, A., Barton, T.K., Beinkhous, A.D.,*

*McCarty, K.S., Moglan, J.A. & McCarty, K.S.:* Apocrine differentiation in human mammary carcinoma. Cancer 1980, 46, 2463-2471.

*Muir, R.:* The evolution of carcinoma of the mamma. J. Pathol. Bact. 1941, 52, 155-171.

*Ozello, L.:* Ultrastructure of intraepithelial carcinomas of the breast. Cancer 1971, 28, 1508-1515.

*Page, D.L., Dupont, W.D., Rogers, L.W. & Landenberger, M.:* Intraductal carcinoma of the breast. Cancer 1982, 49, 751-758.

## Medullary carcinoma with lymphoid stroma infiltration

*Bloom, H.J.G., Richardson, W.W. & Field, J.R.:* Host resistance and survival in carcinoma of breast. Brit. med. J. 1970, 3, 181-188.

*Moore, O.S., Jr. & Foote, F.W.:* The relatively favorable prognosis of medullary carcinoma of the breast. Cancer 1949, 2, 635-642.

*Richardson, W.W.:* Medullary carcinoma of the breast. Brit. J. Cancer 1956, 2, 635.

*Ridolfi, R.L., Rosen, P.P., Port, A., Kinne, D. & Mike, V.:* Medullary carcinoma of the breast. A clinico-pathologic study with 10 year follow-up. Cancer 1977, 40, 1365-1385.

## Lobular carcinoma

*Andersen, J.A.:* The basement membrane and lobular carcinoma in situ of the breast: A light-microscopical study. Acta pathol. microbiol. scand. Sect. A. 1975, 83, 245-250.

*Andersen, J.A.:* Carcinoma lobulare in situ mammae. Thesis, Esbjerg, 1977.

*Andersen, J.A.:* Lobular carcinoma in situ. A long term follow-up in 52 cases. Acta pathol. microbiol. scand. Sect. A. 1974, 82, 519-533.

*Andersen, J.A., Fechner, R.E., Lattes, R., Rosen, P.P. & Toker, C.:* Lobular carcinoma in situ: (lobular neoplasia) of the breast (a symposium). Pathol. Annu. 1980, 15, 193-223.

*Andersen, J.A.:* Lobular carcinoma in situ of the breast. An approach to rational treatment. Cancer 1977, 39, 2597-2602.

*Andersen, J.A. & Vendelboe, M.L.:* Cytoplasmic mucous globules in lobular carcinoma in situ. Diagnosis and prognosis. Amer. J. Surg. Pathol. 1981, 5, 251-255.

*Ashikari, R., Huvos, A.G., Urban, J.A. & Robbins, G.F.:* Infiltrating lobular carcinoma of the breast. Cancer 1973, 31, 110-116.

*Bässler, R.:* Das sogenannte lobuläre Karzinom der Mamma. Pathologie und klinische Konsequenzen. Dtzch. med. Wschr. 1969, 94, 108-113.

*Bässler, R.:* Zur Definition und Dignität des Carcinoma in situ der Brustdrüse. Österr. Z. Onkol. 1975, 2, 125-136.

*Cunningham, L.:* Mastectomy for so-called lobular carcinoma-in-situ. Lancet 1980, I, 106.

*Davis, R.P., Nora, P.F., Kooy, R.G. & Hines, J.R.:* Experience with lobular carcinoma of the breast. Emphasis on recent aspects of management. Arch. Surg. 1979, 114, 485-488.

*Dawson, E.K.:* Carcinoma in the mammary lobule and its origin. Edinburgh med. J. 1933, 40, 57-82.

*Donegan, W.L. & Perez-Mesa, C.M.:* Lobular carcinoma – an indication for elective biopsy of the second breast. Ann. Surg. 1972, 176, 178-187.

*Eusebi, V., Pich, A., Machiorlatti, E. & Bussolati, G.:* Morphofunctional differentiation on the lobular carcinoma of the breast. Histopathology 1977, 1, 301-314.

*Fechner, R.E.:* Ductal carcinoma involving the lobule of the breast. A source of confusion with lobular carcinoma in situ. Cancer 1971, 28, 274-281.

*Fechner, R.E.:* Epithelial alteration in the extralobular ducts of breasts with lobular carcinoma. Arch. Pathol. 1972, 93, 164-171.

*Fechner, R.E.:* Infiltrating lobular carcinoma without lobular carcinoma in situ. Cancer 1972, 29, 1539-1545.

*Fechner, R.E.:* Histologic variants of infiltrating lobular carcinoma of the breast. Hum. Pathol. 1975, 6, 373-378.

*Fechner, R.E.:* Lobular carcinoma in situ in sclerosing adenosis. A potential source of confusion with invasive carcinoma. Amer. J. Surg. Pathol. 1981, 5, 233-239.

*Fisher, E.R., Gregorio, R.M., Redmond, C. & Fisher, B.:* Tubulo-lobular invasive breast carcinoma. A variant of lobular invasive cancer. Hum. Pathol. 1977, 8, 679-683.

*Fisher, E.R. & Fisher, B.:* Lobular carcinoma of the breast. An overview. Ann. Surg. 1978, 185, 377-385.

*Foote, F.W. & Stewart, F.W.:* Lobular carcinoma in situ. A rare form of carcinoma in situ. Amer. J. Pathol. 1941, 17, 491-496.

*Gad, A. & Azzopardi, J.G.:* Lobular carcinoma of the breast. A special variant of mucin-secreting carcinoma. J. clin. Pathol. 1975, 28, 711-716.

*Giordano, J.M. & Klopp, C.T.:* Lobular carcinoma in situ. Incidence and treatment. Cancer 1973, 31, 105-109.

*Godwin, J.T.:* Chronology of lobular carcinoma of the breast. Report of a case. Cancer 1952, 5, 259-266.

*Haagensen, C.D., Lane, N. & Lattes, R.:* Neoplastic proliferation of the epithelium of the mammary lobules. Adenosis, lobular neoplasia, and small cell carcinoma. Surg. clin. North Amer. 1972, 52, 497-524.

*Haagensen, C.D., Lane, N., Lattes, R. & Bodian, C.:* Lobular neoplasia (so called lobular carcinoma in situ) of the breast. Cancer 1978, 42, 737-769.

*Hamperl, H.:* Das lobuläre Carcinoma in situ der Mamma. Histogenese, Wachstum, Übergang in infiltrierendes Karzinom. Dtsch. med. Wschr. 1971, 96, 1585-1588.

*Hamperl, H.:* Zur Kenntnis des sog. Carcinoma lobulare in situ der Mamma. Z. Krebsforsch. 1972, 77, 231-246.

*Hutter, R.V.P., Suyder, R.E., Lucas, J.C., Foote, F.W., Jr. & Farrow, J.H.:* Clinical and pathologic correlation with mammographic findings in lobular carcinoma in situ. Cancer 1969, 23, 826-839.

*Hutter, R.V.P. & Foote, F.W.Jr.:* Lobular carcinoma in situ. Long term follow-up. Cancer 1969, 24, 1081-1085.

*Kahn, L.B. & Webber, B.:* Lobular carcinoma of the breast. A review. Suid-Afrik. Tydskr. Chir. 1974, 12, 51-55.

*Kaufmann, C., Hamperl, H., Baldus, F. & Ki, B.D.:* Das lobuläre Carcinoma in situ der Mamma. Diagnose, Klinik, Therapie. Dtsch. med. Wschr. 1971, 96, 1582-1585.

*Ludwig, A.S., Okagaki, T., Richart, R.M. & Lattes, R.:* Nuclear DNA content of lobular carcinoma in situ of the breast. Cancer 1973, 31, 1553-1560.

*Martinez, V. & Azzopardi, J.G.:* Invasive lobular carcinoma of the breast: incidence and variants. Histopathology 1979, 3, 467-488.

*McDivitt, R.W., Hutter, R.V.P., Foote, F.W., Jr. & Stewart, F.W.:* In situ lobular carcinoma. J. Amer. med. Ass. 1967, 201, 96-100.

*Merino, M.J. & Livolsi, V.A.:* Signet ring carcinoma of the female breast: a clinicopathologic analysis of 24 cases. Cancer 1981, 48, 1830-1837.

*Rosen, P.P., Lieberman, P.H., Braun, D.W., Kosloff, C. & Adair, F.:* Lobular carcinoma in situ of the breast. Detailed analysis of 99 patients with average follow-up of 24 years. Amer. J. Surg. Pathol. 1978, 2, 225-251.

*Schiødt, T.:* Lobulaert carcinoma in situ mammae. En oversigt. Nord. Med. 1971, 85, 45-49.

*Steinbrecher, J.S. & Silverberg, S.G.:* Signet-ring cell carcinoma of the breast. The mucinous variant of infiltrating lobular carcinoma? Cancer 1976, 37, 828-840.

*Toker, C.:* Small cell dysplasia and in-situ carcinoma of the mammary ducts and lobules. J. Pathol. 1974, 114, 47-52.

*Toker, C. & Goldberg, J.D.:* The small cell lesion of mammary ducts and lobules. Pathol. Annu. 1977, 12, 217-249.

*Tulusan, A.H., Egger, H., Schneider, M.L. & Willgeroth, F.:* A contribution to the natural history of breast cancer. IV. Lobular carcinoma in situ and its relation to breast cancer. Arch. Gynecol. 1982, 231, 219-226.

*Warner, N.E.:* Lobular carcinoma of the breast. Cancer 1969, 23, 840-846.

*Wheeler, J.E., Enterline, H.T., Roseman, J.M. Tomasulo, J.P., McIdvaine, C.H., Fitts, W.T. & Kirshenbaum, J.:* Lobular carcinoma in situ of the breast. Long-term follow-up. Cancer 1974, 34, 554-563.

*Wheeler, J.E. & Enterline, H.T.:* Lobular carcinoma of the breast in situ and infiltrating. Pathol. Annu. 1976, 11, 161-188.

## Special types of carcinoma

*Aboumrad, M.H., Horn, R.C., Jr. & Fine, G.:* Lipid-secreting mammary carcinoma. Cancer 1963, 16, 521-525.

*Akhtar, M., Robinson, C., Ashraf Ali, M. & Godwin, J.T.:* Secretory carcinoma of the breast in adults. Light and electron microscopic study of three cases with review of the literature. Cancer 1983, 51, 2245-2254.

*Anthony, P.P. & James, P.D.:* Adenoid cystic carcinoma of the breast: prevalence, diagnostic criteria and histogenesis. J. clin. Pathol. 1975, 28, 647-655.

*Azzopardi, J.G., Muretto, P., Goddeeris, P., Eusebi, V. & Lauweryns, J.M.:* "Carcinoid" tumours of the breast: the morphological spectrum of argyrophil carcinomas. Histopathology 1982, 6, 549-569.

*van Bogaert, L.-J. & Maldaque.P.:* Histologic variants of lipid-secreting carcinoma of the breast. Virch. Arch. Abt. A. 1977, 375, 345-353.

*Bässler, R.:* Pathologie der weiblichen Genital- und Mammatumoren in Kindesalter und Adoleszenz. Gynäkologe 1973, 6, 49-65.

*Capella, C., Eusebi, V., Mann, B. & Azzopardi, J.G.:* Endocrine differentiation in mucoid carcinoma of the breast. Histopathology 1980, 4, 613-630.

*Cavanzo, F.J. & Taylor, H.B.:* Adenoid cystic carcinoma of the breast. An analysis of 21 cases. Cancer 1969, 24, 740-745.

*Clayton, F., Sibley, R., Ordonez, N.G. & Hanssen, G.:* Argyrophilic breast carcinomas. Evidence of lactational differentiation. Amer. J. Surg. Pathol. 1982, 6, 323-333.

*Devitt, P.G.:* Carcinoid tumour of the breast. Brit. med. J. 1978, 2, 327.

*Elsner, B.:* Adenoid cystic carcinoma of the breast. Review of the literature and clinico-pathologic study of seven patients. Path. Europ. 1970, 5, 357-364.

*Fetissof, F., Dubois, M.P., Arbeille-Brassart, B., Lansac, J. & Jobard, P.:* Argyrophilic cells in mammary carcinoma. Hum. Pathol. 1983, 14, 127-134.

*Friedman, B.A. & Oberman, H.A.:* Adenoid cystic carcinoma of the breast. Amer. J. clin. Pathol. 1970, 54, 1-14.

*Harris, M.:* Pseudoadenoid cystic carcinoma of the breast. Arch. Pathol. lab. Med. 1977, 101, 307-309.

*Hjorth, S., Magnusson, P.H. & Blomquist, P.:* Adenoid cystic carcinoma of the breast. Report of a case in a male and review of the literature. Acta chir. scand. 1977, 143, 155-158.

*Koss, L.G., Brannan, C.D. & Ashikari, R.:* Histologic and ultrastructural features of adenoid-cystic carcinoma of the breast.

Cancer 1970, 26, 1271-1279.

*McDivitt, R.W. & Stewart, F.W.:* Breast carcinoma in children. J. Amer. med. Ass. 1966, 195, 144-146.

*Quizilbash, A.H., Patterson, M.C. & Oliveira, K.F.:* Adenoid cystic carcinoma of the breast. Light and electron microscopy and a brief review of the literature. Arch. Pathol. lab. Med. 1977, 101, 302-306.

*Ramos, C.V. & Taylor, H.B.:* Lipid-rich carcinoma of the breast. A clinico-pathologic analysis of 13 examples. Cancer 1974, 33, 812-819.

*Rosen, P.P.:* Multinucleated mammary stromal giant cells. A benign lesion that simulates invasive carcinoma. Cancer 1979, 44, 1305-1308.

*Sugano, I., Nagao, K., Kondo, Y., Nabeshima, S. & Murakami, S.:* Cytologic and ultra-structural studies of a rare breast carcinoma with osteoclast-like giant cells. Cancer 1983, 52, 74-78.

*Tavassoli, F.A. & Norris, H.J.:* Secretory carcinoma of the breast. Cancer 1980, 45, 2404-2413.

*Taxy, J.B., Tischler, A.S., Insalaco, S.J. & Battifora, H.:* "Carcinoid" tumor of the breast. A variant of conventional breast cancer? Hum. Pathol. 1981, 12, 170-179.

*Wilson, W.B. & Spell, J.P.:* Adenoid cystic carcinoma of the breast. A case with occurrence and regional metastases. Ann. Surg. 1967, 166, 861-864.

## Special problems in carcinoma (combined types, bilateral and occult carcinoma, regression of carcinoma, metastases).

*Berge, T. & Östberg, G.:* Bilateral carcinoma of the female breast. Acta chir. scand. 1974, 140, 27-32.

*Cowen, P.N.:* Recognition of intraduct carcinoma. Letter to the Editor. J. Clin. Pathol. 1980, 33, 797.

Crile, G.: Multicentric breast cancer. The incidence of new cancers in the homolateral breast after partial mastectomy. Cancer 1975, 35, 475-477.

Egan, R.L.: Bilateral breast carcinomas. Role of mammography. Cancer 1976, 38, 931-938.

Engelbreth-Holm, J.: Om hyppigheden af dobbelsidig brystkræft og om brystkræftens sammentræf med andre kræftformer. Ugeskr. Læger 1942, 104, 456-461.

Hutter, R.V.P. & Kim, D.U.: The problem of multiple lesions of the breast. Cancer 1971, 28, 1591-1607.

Jackson, J.G. & Orr, J.W.: The ducts of carcinomatous breasts, with particular reference to connective tissue changes. J. Pathol. Bact. 1957, 74, 265-273.

Kesseler, H.J., Grier, W.R.N., Seildman, I. & McIlveen, S.J.: Bilateral primary breast cancer. J. Am. med. Ass. 1976, 236, 278-280.

Kilgore, A.R., Bell, H.G. & Ahlquist, R.E.: Cancer in the second breast. Amer. J. Surg. 1956, 92, 156-161.

Lagios, M.D.: Multicentricity of breast carcinoma demonstrated by routine correlated serial subgross and radiographic examination. Cancer 1977, 40, 1726-1734.

Leis, H.P.: Selective, elective, prophylactic contralateral mastectomy. Cancer 1971, 28, 956-961.

Lewison, E.F. & Neto, A.S.: Bilateral breast cancer at the Johns Hopkins Hospital. A discussion of the dilemma of contralateral breast cancer. Cancer 1971, 28, 1297-1301.

Linell, F., Palmer, B. & Ringberg, A.: Det kontralaterala bröstet vid bröstcancer. Problem vid rekonstruktionskirurgi. Läkaresällskapets Riksstämma, Stockholm, 1981.

Muir, R. & Aitkenhead, A.C.: The healing of intra-duct carcinoma of the mamma. J.

Pathol. Bact. 1934, 38, 117-127.

Qualheim, R.E. & Gall, E.A.: Breast carcinoma with multiple sites of origin. Cancer 1957, 10, 460-468.

Ringberg, A., Palmer, B. & Linell, F.: The contralateral breast at reconstructive surgery after breast cancer operation – A histopathological study. Breast Cancer Res. Treatment 1982, 2, 151-161.

Robbins, G.F. & Berg, J.W.: Bilateral primary breast cancers. A prospective clinicopathological study. Cancer 1964, 17, 1501-1527.

Rosen, P.P.: Coexistent lobular carcinoma in situ and intraductal carcinoma in a single lobular-duct unit. Amer. J. Surg. Pathol. 1980, 4, 241-246.

Schwartz, G.F., Patchefsky, A.S., Feig, S.A., Schaber, G.S. & Schwartz, A.B.: Clinically occult breast carcinoma. Multicentricity and implications for treatment. Ann. Surg. 1980, 191, 8-12.

Urban, J.A., Papachriston, D. & Taylor, J.: Bilateral breast cancer. Biopsy of the opposite breast. Cancer 1977, 40, 1960-1973.

Webber, B.L., Heise, H., Neifeld, J.P. & Costa, J.: Risk of subsequent contralateral breast carcinoma in a population of patients with in-situ breast carcinoma. Cancer 1981, 47, 2928-2932.

# References to Chapters 7 and 16.
## Mesenchymal tumors

Angiosarcoma of the breast. Editorial. Amer. J. Surg. Pathol. 1981, 5, 679-680.

Donnell, R.M., Rosen, P.P., Lieberman, Ph.D., Kaufman, R.J., Kay, S., Braun, D.W. & Kinne, D.W.: Angiosarcoma and other vascular tumors of the breast. Pathologic analysis as a guide to prognosis. Amer. J. Surg. Pathol. 1981, 5, 629-642.

Hajdu, S.I., Espinosa, M.H. & Robbins, G.F.: Recurrent cystosarcoma phyllodes. A clinicopathologic study of 32 cases. Cancer

1976, 38, 1402-1406.

*Hamperl, H.:* Hämangioma der menschlichen Mamma. Geburtsh. Frauenheilk. 1973, 33, 13-17.

*Hamperl, H. & Warambo, W.:* Leiomyosarcoma of the breast originating from myothelium (myoepithelium). J. Pathol. 1974, 114, 89-92.

*Kahn, L.B., Uys, C.J., Dale, J. & Rutherfoord, F.:* Carcinoma of the breast with metaplasia to chondrosarcoma: a light and electron microscopic study. Histopathology 1978, 2, 93-106.

*Mambo, U.C., Burke, J.S. & Butler, J.J.:* Primary malignant lymphomas of the breast. Cancer 1977, 39, 2033-2040.

*Menon, M. & van Velthoven, P.C.M.:* Liposarcoma of the breast. A case report. Arch. Pathol. 1974, 98, 370-372.

*Miettinen, M., Letho, V.-P. & Virtanen, I.:* Postmastectomy angiosarcoma (Stewart-Treves syndrome). Light-microscopic, immunohistological and ultrastructural characteristics of two cases. Amer. J. Surg. Pathol. 1983, 7, 329-339.

*Norris, H.J. & Taylor, H.B.:* Relationship of histologic features to behaviour of cystosarcoma phyllodes. Analysis of ninety-four cases. Cancer 1969, 20, 2090-2099.

*Rhodes, R.H., Frankel, K.A., Davis, L. & Tatter, D.:* Metastatic cystosarcoma phyllodes. A report of 2 cases presenting with neurological symptoms. Cancer 1978, 41, 1179-1189.

*Rosen, P.P. & Ridolfi, R.L.:* The perilobular hemangioma. Amer. J. Clin. Pathol. 1977, 68, 21-23.

*Shore, J.H.:* Hemangiosarcoma of the breast. J. Pathol. Bact. 1957, 74, 289-293.

*Steingaszner, L.C., Enzinger, F.M. & Taylor, H.B.:* Hemangiosarcoma of the breast. Cancer 1965, 18, 352-361.

*Toker, C., Tang, C.-K., Whitely, J.F., Berkeiser, S.M. & Rackman, R.:* Benign spindle cell breast tumor. Cancer 1981, 48, 1615-1622.

# References to Chapters 8 and 17.
## *Mammillary diseases*

*Bhagavan, B.S., Patchefsky, A. & Koss, L.G.:* Florid subareolar duct papillomatosis (nipple adenoma) and mammary carcinoma: report of three cases. Hum. Pathol. 1973, 4, 289-295.

*Citoler, P. & Zippel, H.-H.:* Carcinombefall der Mamilla bei Mammacarcinomen. Gynäkologie 1974, 7, 186-189.

*Congdon, G.H. & Dockerty, M.B.:* Malignant lesions of the nipple exclusive of Paget's disease. Surg. Gynecol. Obstet. 1956, 103, 185-192.

*Davis, A.B. & Patchefsky, A.S.:* Basal cell carcinoma of the nipple. Case report and review of the literature. Cancer 1977, 40, 1780-1781.

*Gould, V.E. & Snyder, R.W.:* Ultrastructural features of papillomatosis and carcinoma of nipple ducts. The significance of myoepithelial cells and basal lamina in benign "questionable" and malignant lesions. Pathol. Annu. 1974, 9, 441-469.

*Gudjónsdóttir, Á., Hägerstrand, I. & Östberg, G.:* Adenoma of the nipple with carcinomatous development. Acta pathol. microbiol. scand. Sect. A. 1971, 79, 676-680.

*Jones, D.B.:* Florid papillomatosis of the nipple ducts. Cancer 1955, 8, 315-319.

*Muir, R.:* The pathogenesis of Paget's disease of the nipple and associated lesions. Brit. J. Surg. 1935, 22, 728-735.

*Muir, R.:* Further observations on Paget's disease of the nipple. J. Pathol. Bact. 1939, 49, 299-312.

*Perzin, K.H. & Lattes, R.:* Papillary adenoma of the nipple (florid papillomatosis, adenoma, adenomatosis). A clinicopathologic study. Cancer 1972, 29, 996-1009.

Taylor, H.B. & Robertson, A.G.: Adenomas of the nipple. Cancer 1965, 18, 995-1002.

Toker, C.: Clear cells of the nipple epidermis. Cancer 1970, 25, 601-610.

## References to Chapters 9 and 18.
### Diseases of the male breast

Andersen, J.A. & Gram, J.B.: Male breast at autopsy. Acta pathol. microbiol. immunol. scand. Sect. A. 1982, 90, 191-197.

Andersen, J.A. & Gram, J.B.: Gynecomasty. Histological aspects in a surgical material. Acta pathol. microbiol. immunol. scand. Sect. A. 1982, 90, 185-190.

Berge, T.: Metastases of the male breast. Acta pathol. microbiol. scand. Sect. A. 1971, 79, 491-496.

Berge, T. & Lundberg, S.: Cancer in Malmö 1958-1969. An autopsy study. Acta pathol. microbiol. scand. Sect. A. 1977, Suppl. 220, Munksgaard, Copenhagen.

Scheike, O.: Male breast cancer. Factors influencing prognosis. Brit. J. Cancer 1974, 30, 261-271.

Scheike, O.: Male breast cancer. Acta pathol. microbiol. scand. Sect. A. Suppl, 251, Munksgaard, Copenhagen, 1975.

Sirtori, C. & Veronesi, U.: Gynecomastia. A review of 218 cases. Cancer 1957, 10, 645-654.

Taxy, J.B.: Tubular carcinoma of the male breast. Cancer 1975, 36, 462-465.

## References to Chapters 10 and 19.
### Varia

Bogomoletz, W.V., Boulenger, E. & Simatos, A.: Infiltrating fibromatosis of the breast. J. clin. Pathol. 1981, 34, 30-34.

Hamperl, H.: The myothelia (myoepithelial cells). Normal state; regressive changes; hyperplasia; tumors. Curr. Topics Pathol. 1970, 53, 161-220.

Jönsson, G., Linell, F. & Sandblom, P.: Subcutaneous cords on the trunk. Acta chir. scand. 1955, 108, 351-367.

Rosen, Y., Papasozomenos, S.C. & Gardner, B.: Fibromatosis of the breast. Cancer 1978, 41, 1409-1413.

Sheth, M.T., Hathway, D. & Petrelli, M.: Pleomorphic adenoma ("mixed" tumor) of human female breast mimicking carcinoma clinico-radiologically. Cancer 1978, 41, 659-665.

# Subject Index

Lobular
    atypia, cribrous   116-119
    neoplasia   200-203
Lymph nodes
    elastosis in   242-243
    examination of   15-16
    metastasis   154-155, 158-159, 240-243
    sarcoid reaction in   64-65
    technique of investigation of   15-16
Lymphadenosis benigna cutis   34, 268-269
Lymphangiography   72-73
Lymphatic spread of carcinoma   186-187
Lymphoedema   33
Lymphoid stroma infiltration in car-
cinoma   196-199

# M

Macromastia
    in pregnancy   18, 52-53
Macroscopic examination   15-17
    specimen radiography   15
Male breast   35
    carcinoma in   35
    gynecomastia   35, 270-273
    metastasis in   35
Mammary
    duct ectasia, see Ductectasia
    dysplasia, see Cystic breast disease
Mammilla, see also Nipple
    adenocarcinoma of   34, 266-267
    adenoma of   34, 262-265
    florid adenomatosis of   34, 262-265
    normal structure   38-39
Mammography
    calcifications in   23, 96-99
    carcinoma types in   29
    retraction in   120-121
Mastitis
    chronic   62-63
    foreign bodies and   70-73
    granulomatous   64-65
    necrosis in   21
    obliterative   68-69
    plasma cell   66-71

retention   66-71
tuberculous   21
unspecific   62-63
Mastopathy, see Cystic breast disease
Mastoplasia, see Cystic breast disease
Menarche
    changes in the breast during   18
Menopause
    involution of the breast   54-55
Menstrual cycle
    changes in breast during   19, 46-47
Metaplasia
    adipose   54-55
    apocrine   92-93
Metastases
    elastin formation in   242-243
    in comedo carcinoma   240-241
    in lobular carcinoma   242-243
    in tubular carcinoma   154-155, 240-241
    unusual forms of   240-243
Microglandular adenosis   24, 108-109
Mondor's disease   36
Mucin
    formation in carcinoma   190-195
Myoepithelioma   276-279
Myothelium   38-39
    mimicking nerve invasion   40-41
    normal   38-39
    proliferation in sclerosing adenosis   100-107
    islands of   40-41
Myxomatous stroma in fibroadenoma   76-77

# N

Narben, strahlige, see Radial scar
Necrosis
    due to anticoagulants   21
    in mastitis   21
    infarction, hemorrhagic   21
Nerve invasion   40-41
    myothelium, mimicking   40-41
    in sclerosing adenosis   40-41
Nipple, see Mammilla
Nodular fasciitis   278-281